GETTING
=IN=
SHAPE

David Denison is professor of clinical physiology at the Brompton Hospital, an international authority on lung function, and a keen advocate of the need for preventative medicine.

Gay Search is a writer and broadcaster and regularly contributes to magazines, radio and television. She is author of SURVIVING DIVORCE: A HANDBOOK FOR MEN and (with David Roper) THE PINEAPPLE DANCE BOOK.

GETTING
=IN=
SHAPE

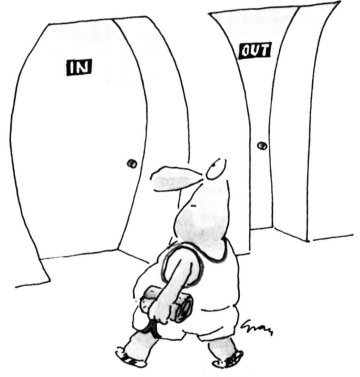

GAY SEARCH and DAVID DENISON
ILLUSTRATED BY GRAY JOLLIFFE

NEW ENGLISH LIBRARY

First published in Great Britain in 1988 by
New English Library, Mill Road, Dunton Green, Sevenoaks, Kent.

Editorial office: 47 Bedford Square, London WC1B 3DP.

British Library Cataloguing in Publication Data

Search, Gay
   Getting in shape.
   1. Physical fitness
   I. Title   II. Denison, David
   613.7   RA781

ISBN: 0 450 39939 7

Typeset by Rowland Phototypesetting Ltd
Bury St Edmunds, Suffolk
Printed in Great Britain by
T J Press (Padstow) Ltd, Padstow, Cornwall

Designed by Jeremy Dixon

CONTENTS

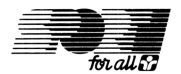

Foreword by John Smith, Chairman of the Sports Council

As a nation, we are much more health conscious today than we were ten years ago. Exercise is now both popular and fashionable as many health centres, dance studios and fitness complexes have sprung up to service the growing demand.

Despite this boom in mass participation, a lot of people still do not take part in any form of exercise and this book is aimed at them.

Getting in Shape helps the non-participant take that first (and hardest) step towards an active lifestyle. The experiences of the project volunteers prove that it is possible to get fit safely and relatively painlessly without sacrificing too much leisure time.

This book tells the story of the *Getting in Shape* participants – why they volunteered, what their training involved and what effects this had on their bodies, their self image and their lifestyle.

More importantly, *Getting in Shape* offers the non-participant an easy-to-follow fitness programme. The Sports Council welcomes this publication and its contribution to promoting 'Sport for All'.

INTRODUCTION

This book began as a study of the effects of a 'get-fit' programme on a group of people who were thirty years old or more, felt they were unfit and wanted to do something to put that right. At the end of a year of training which was not desperately rigorous or tiring, almost all of them felt very much better. They were physically fitter, but also much more able to cope with mental and emotional challenges as well, which is one of the good things about getting fit. The psychological benefits and the considerable increases in mental and physical endurance far out-weigh the physical improvements measured in fitness clinics.

The study took some months to design and organise, another eighteen months to run, and a further year to analyse and report. It is very gratifying to discover that the scientific research does make a compelling case for the benefits of exercise. Everyone who took part in the project hopes that this book will encourage others to improve their physical condition secure in the knowledge that their efforts are based on a programme that has been scientifically tested.

We are deeply grateful to everyone who took part in the GETTING IN SHAPE project and both of us would like to make sure that credit goes where it is due, namely to:

a) The participants, who prefer to remain nameless but were marvellously co-operative and made it all possible.

b) Bev Risman, Tom McNab and Sandy Larvan who prepared the training schedules; Gray Jolliffe who illustrated them; Cathy Crilley, Val Day, Ian Evans, James Godber, John Goody, Joyce Goody, Nick Gray, Patrick Green, Brenda Green, Debbie Hoyle, Carole Humphryes, Rodney Lewis, Jim Miller, Hilda Nyman, Alec Randall, Bobby Randall, Mick Rankin, Diana Rayfield, John Routledge, Laurie Thompson, Bernie Tuck, John Walker and Wendy Wood who were the dedicated volunteer trainers on whom the project hinged.

c) Geoffrey Cannon (then a journalist for the *Sunday Times*) and Will Chapman (then and now a leading light of the London

Road Runners) who conceived the original idea and brought it to the West London Institute and then to the Brompton Hospital where it 'took shape'.

d) The National Heart and Chest Hospitals, the West London Institute of Higher Education, the Sports Council, the Health Education Council, the *Sunday Times* and the participants, who funded the study.

e) Will Chapman and Jane Howarth, who administered the day by day organisation of the whole trial with great calm and tact.

f) Doctors Michael Morgan, Andrew Peacock, Andrew Bush, Bob Green and Paul Oldershaw, who organised and ran the medical examinations; and Doctors Durrald Barham, Les Galaska, Ben Gilfeather, James Sainsbury, Sidney Scott, Andrew Surawy, David Wilks and Martin Wolfson, who were on hand to give sports medicine advice through the year.

g) Malcolm Emery, Dr Nick Walters, Guy Selwood, Mark Saunders, Alison Lyne, Sue McNuff and Debbie Albutt, who conducted the exercise tests, at the West London Institute.

h) Dr Hadi Al-Hillawi, Hazel Belfield-Smith, Derek Cramer, Sonia Burke, Simon Johnson, Susannah Greenberg, Jan Ball, Simon Ward, Haab Birdi, Peter Longbourne, Pam Hancox, Dr Mike Morgan, Tom Sopwith and Dr Andrew Peacock, who made the lung function studies and body shape measurements.

i) John Lovesey and Alistair Brett of the *Sunday Times*, Bev Stephens and Pauline Ashworth of the Sports Council; and Cathy Crilley and Dr Alan Maryon-Davies of the Health Education Council, who gave us continued support and management advice.

j) Hazel Belfield-Smith, who interviewed the participants at the end of the study and together with Dr Al-Hillawi wrote large parts of the formal report.

k) Rosemary Scott and Julie Anagnostou for the vast amount of secretarial work involved.

David Denison and Gay Search

1
THE PROJECT

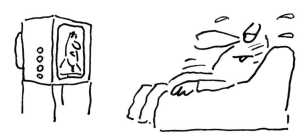

It's undeniable that we as a nation are much more health-conscious than we were ten or even five years ago. Health and fitness are now the staple diet of radio and television programmes as well as books, newspapers and magazines, and hardly a week goes by without some new statistic being unearthed. Heart and lung disease, for example, is now known to be responsible for half of all deaths in this country, for half the time spent in hospital and for half of all working days lost. It's also known that in many cases these diseases are, to some extent, self-inflicted through smoking, poor diet and lack of exercise and, therefore, preventable. And so we try to give up smoking, are more careful about what we eat, and think about taking up some form of exercise.

Certainly the last few years have seen an exercise boom. Most towns now boast gymnasiums, dance centres and jogging clubs, and there are more and more 'citizen races' which attract thousands of people who are running for their health and for fun, not for the glory of winning.

But there are still thousands more who don't get beyond the thinking stage. You know by the way you're breathing hard when you get to the top of the stairs that you are unfit, but you're daunted by the prospect of doing something about it – memories of school perhaps and being humiliated by the games teacher, or fear that you really have left it too late and that getting back into shape will be just too painful – and you find any number of excuses. You haven't got time; it's dangerous at your age to start taking violent exercise; it's just a fad – your grandfather weighed sixteen stone, smoked eighty a day, the only exercise he ever took was the two-minute walk to the pub on the corner and he lived to be ninety!

But you *can* get fit, safely, relatively painlessly, and without it disrupting your life, as the experience of the GETTING IN SHAPE participants proves conclusively. The vast majority of the ordinary, unfit, middle-aged men and women who took part in the project – many of whom had some, if not all, of the reservations mentioned above – not only improved their fitness, but thoroughly enjoyed exercising and felt their overall sense of well-being, their self-confidence and zest for living enhanced to a degree that no one had foreseen.

GETTING IN SHAPE tells their story – why they volunteered; what they went through in terms of training and testing; what it did to their bodies, their way of life, their self-image – and based on the lessons learnt, offers you a programme for getting in shape.

GETTING IN SHAPE had its origins in the first London Marathon in 1981. Geoffrey Cannon, then a *Sunday Times* journalist and more recently co-author of *Dieting Makes You Fat* and *The Food Scandal*, ran in the marathon, and wrote an article for *Running* magazine about his experiences of training on his own. He ended by asking any readers who liked the idea of training in a group for the next London Marathon to write in. Fifty people responded, only six of whom had run a marathon before. They met in Hyde Park one Saturday and since their target was the '82 London Marathon, they called themselves 'London 82/50'.

Since they didn't all live in London, they formed local groups and ran together once a week and went for a drink together afterwards. A few people dropped out but others joined and eventually clubs were formed, like the Stragglers in Bushey Park near Richmond and eventually the Serpentine Running Club in Hyde Park.

Even before the '82 Marathon was run – with 'London 82/50' well represented – Cannon was so impressed with the results that he came up with the idea of taking complete beginners, as out of shape as possible, and training them in twenty weeks for the *Sunday Times* Fun Run – 4 kilometres/2.5 miles – in Hyde Park that autumn.

His article in the May issue of *Running* magazine announcing 'Fun Runner '82' produced over 100 volunteers. Sixty-four were finally chosen and divided into groups under the leadership of 'London 82/50' members who had got so much enjoyment and benefit from running themselves that they wanted to spread the word.

Two sports physiologists from Chester College, Kevin Sykes and Ted Charlesworth, had developed a relatively simple fitness-monitoring programme to check body fat, blood pressure, cardiovascular fitness and lung efficiency. They agreed to test the volunteers before they started training, half-way through and again at the end.

The project was a great success. Not only did two-thirds of the original sixty-four finish the training and take part in the Fun Run, but the effects on their fitness were very encouraging. Although the men lost only 7 lb in weight on average and the women 4 lb, the percentage of body fat dropped on average 25% and 12% respectively, and there was a significant healthy drop in average blood pressure levels too.

The participants also filled in questionnaires designed by a research psychologist to see whether it is possible to determine objectively if exercise affects mood or mental state. The results showed that the fitter people are, the higher their intelligence scores, and the more emotionally stable, self-assured, relaxed and non-conformist they are likely to be. 'Fun Runner '82' was such a success, not only in terms of improved fitness, but in terms of sheer enjoyment, too, that Cannon decided to try and set up a similar project on a nation-wide basis under the sponsorship of the *Sunday Times*.

For various reasons it proved impractical, but then a group of people came together by chance: Will Chapman, a member of 'London 82/50' who had become increasingly involved in organising 'citizen races' in his spare time; Malcolm Emery, then senior lecturer in physiology at the West London Institute of Higher Education; and David Denison, professor of clinical physiology at the Brompton Hospital and an international authority on lung function.

David Denison readily agreed to oversee the scientific aspects of the project partly because one of the Brompton's long-term aims is to develop preventive medicine, but mainly because such a project offered a unique opportunity for himself and his colleagues to collect data on the effects of exercise on normal, healthy people – something that hospitals understandably find very difficult to get. Astonishingly, in spite of all that has been written and in spite of many widely held beliefs, there was no conclusive medical evidence that for the average man and woman exercise would improve the workings of the cardio-vascular system and thereby lessen the risk of heart or lung disease. Research had been carried out into the effects of exercise on people already suffering from heart disease, depression or obesity and on super-fit, young athletes, but what it did to the vast majority of us, no one really knew. So, with Will Chapman as full-time administrative director, GETTING IN SHAPE was underway.

Although the original plan was that the training should be basically jogging, like 'Fun Runner '82', the team realised that it was a unique opportunity to test theories about the effects of different types of exercise, as well as studying the general effect. The sports physiologists at the West London Institute already knew that, although all athletes need the same amount of oxygen to produce the same amount of work, they use it in different ways. Those in explosive events like sprinting and jumping where the muscles work without oxygen – anaerobic exercise – use it quite differently from those in endurance events like long-distance running, cycling or swimming where the muscles need a steady supply of oxygen to function – aerobic exercise. They knew too that it was due to the different types of muscle that predominate in the two groups of athletes – white or 'fast twitch' in the anaerobes, and red or 'slow twitch' among the aerobes. What they didn't know, though, was whether the predominance of one muscle type was genetic or acquired as the result of training. They hoped that by subjecting ordinary, unfit people to the two different types of training they might come up with the answer.

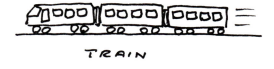

TRAIN

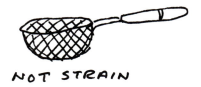

NOT STRAIN

The plan was to recruit 100 men and women, roughly between the ages of thirty and fifty-five, who believed themselves to be unfit and wanted to do something about it. They would be divided into pairs, as closely matched as possible for sex, age, height and weight and asked to train under supervision for about two hours a week for a year, one of each pair doing aerobic training – walking, swimming, cycling, as well as jogging – to develop endurance, and the other doing anaerobic training – press-ups, squat thrusts and so on – to develop flexibility and strength. They would undergo physiological tests at four-monthly intervals and at the end of the year the team would be able to compare the effects of the different kinds of training.

Although the GETTING IN SHAPE doctors, physiologists and trainers would be giving their services free, other costs – administration, hire of sports halls and so on – had to be covered. The Sports Council contributed £15,000, the Health Education Council £6,325 and the *Sunday Times* £2,500. It was decided to charge the participants £100 each, which the team felt was good value considering one set of physiological tests alone would normally cost £90 and they were to be tested four times.

On September 19th 1982, Geoffrey Cannon's article announcing GETTING IN SHAPE appeared in the *Sunday Times*, inviting readers who felt they were unfit and were prepared to commit themselves to a year of training and tests to write to Will Chapman for an application form.

The first letter, hand-delivered, dropped through Will Chapman's letter-box at 9.30 that morning, and the trickle soon became a flood. By the closing date, he had received almost 1,500 applications, just over a third from women, and the overwhelming majority – 86% – expressing interest in aerobic rather than anaerobic training.

Although the original idea had been to offer a choice of aerobic training – swimming, cycling and walking as well as jogging – it soon became clear that it would be virtually impossible to find the right sort of volunteers to act as trainers in all those sports, and as 'Fun Runner '82' had demonstrated, the trainers would be crucial to the success of the project. Besides, the non-medical members of the team felt that with a few people doing a wide range of activities, the group element which they believed to be vitally important in keeping people motivated to carry on training would be lost. So aerobic training became jogging. Rather than recruit as trainers qualified physical education instructors who had never been unfit in their lives, the team decided to recruit relative beginners who were very keen to share their new-found enthusiasm for exercise with other people but for whom the memories of being unfit and struggling to run more than a few yards were still very fresh.

Bev Risman, former England rugby fly half and now senior lecturer in physical education science at the West London Institute, was invited to prepare training schedules for the aerobic and anaerobic groups. Although Risman had spent a large part of his working life dealing with young super-fit athletes, he had worked in adult education running courses for older, unfit people – experience that stood him in good stead.

A simple warm-up routine was devised for both groups to get the heart and lungs working harder and to warm up and stretch the muscles. Risman set out to make the anaerobic programme, designed to strengthen all the major muscle groups in the body and improve flexibility, as simple as possible so that the participants, who would be exercising at home on their own for much of the time, could follow it with a minimum of supervision.

Since few of the trainers had experience of anaerobics they had to acquaint themselves thoroughly with all the exercises and the proper techniques. 'Although the exercises themselves are very simple – push-ups, sit-ups, step-ups and so on – it was vital that people did them properly and didn't inadvertently find ways of cheating. Once they'd got the exercises right it was very important that the trainers didn't let them rush ahead too fast.'

The planning of the aerobic training programme was more of a joint effort. 'No one had more experience of training people who hadn't exercised for years than the "Fun Runner '82" trainers,' said Will Chapman,' so we knew better than the fitness experts what was realistic and what wasn't. It's hard for people who've always been fit and are used to dealing with athletes to accept that it is not actually possible for some people to jog for more than a few minutes when they first start. In the end they came round to our way of thinking.'

Motivation was obviously a key factor, something Bev Risman had to bear very much in mind. 'In my experience, the drop-out rate in exercise programmes, whether it's circuit training or aerobic dancing, is tremendously high – up to 75% within the first month. With GETTING IN SHAPE we couldn't afford to let that happen because we needed to collect data on a significant number of people. We weren't too worried about the aerobic groups, but anaerobic training does get boring, so we did stress to the trainers that they had to find ways of keeping their groups motivated.'

In the meantime, everyone who responded to the original *Sunday Times* article was sent an application form asking for details of their life style – whether they smoked and drank – and of their own and their family's medical history. They were also asked to give permission for their GP to be approached and to express a preference for one type of training. The team wound up with over 800 applications for the 100 places, so it decided to increase the number and select 180 people on the basis that some of them would drop out when they actually had to hand over the £100, leaving it with approximately 150 participants.

The actual selection was done by computer. Will Chapman wrote a programme asking it to select pairs – one aerobe and one anaerobe – as closely matched as possible for sex, age, height and weight, with a tolerance of three years, two inches and five pounds respectively.

'The men were no problem. There were enough who had opted for both types of training to produce forty-five pairs. The women were more difficult. Very few had opted for anaerobics because I think they imagined it would be weight training and they'd wind up looking like shot-putters. I contacted a few aerobes who hadn't been selected and asked if they would be prepared to do anaerobics instead. If they didn't seem keen I didn't push it. No point in asking people to do something they're not happy about.

'The only other tinkering I did with the computer's pairings was to try and broaden the spectrum a little. In the first sweep for instance, it produced lots of men who were 5'10" and 11 stone. We felt the sample should match the population at large more closely so we included a few pairs who were very big and very small.'

180 people were invited to the first meeting in October, most of whom turned up. They were told what the project would involve: attending a group-training session once a week at one of seven centres in the London area, and going for a drink with members of their group afterwards; training on their own two or three times a week according to their schedule; keeping a training diary; attending four testing sessions at the Brompton Hospital and the West London Institute before they started, after four months, after eight months and at the end of the year. They were invited to pay the £100 and told that, provided they passed a preliminary medical, they were accepted.

'As we'd expected,' Will Chapman said, 'some people dropped out at that point, but there were quite a few couples present from which only one person had been accepted. Some of the unsuccessful partners asked if they could join in and since it made sense from a motivational point of view to have them both exercising, we accepted them. It meant a bit of juggling with the pairings we'd already done, and half a dozen extra people who hadn't been accepted first time round were brought in to fill the gaps.'

The participants were told they all had a 'twin', but not who he or she was. The team felt that if people knew their twin had dropped out, or discovered that he or she was making much more dramatic progress, their motivation might be adversely affected.

176 people underwent medicals at the Brompton Hospital, and only two were found to have problems serious enough to prevent them from taking part. They were both women and both had heart conditions about which they hadn't previously known.

By the beginning of May 1983 there were 174 volunteers, training manuals in their hands, kitted out in tracksuits and training shoes and having undergone the first series of tests, eager to start.

2

PEOPLE LIKE YOU

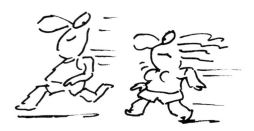

The 174 people who embarked on GETTING IN SHAPE were indeed a mixed bunch. They ranged in age from thirty to fifty-nine, and included almost every conceivable shape and size – from 5'0" to 6'4" and from 7 stone 11 lb to 18 stone. As you might expect of *Sunday Times* readers, many of them had executive or managerial jobs, were in the professions, or were self-employed. There were lawyers, teachers, nurses and other health professionals (though only one GP, who dropped out very early on), company directors, chartered accountants, journalists, artists, house-wives, a bank manager, a fashion designer, an Oscar-winning screen writer and an income tax inspector. Most of them lived in the Greater London area, though some travelled in from the home counties – Berkshire, Bedfordshire, the Essex coast – and one man, a telecommunications engineer who was posted to Rotterdam soon after the project started, commuted back at least once a month to attend group sessions and all the medical tests.

Although all the participants considered themselves unfit – that was the reason for getting involved in GETTING IN SHAPE in the first place – the levels of fitness actually varied quite con-siderably. Some people who had been very active in their teens and twenties but who had done nothing in the way of sport or exercise in recent years now felt themselves to be appallingly unfit by comparison. Other people who had done as little sport as possible at school – 'I spent all my time trying to avoid the games mistress's eye' – and nothing at all since, knew they weren't super-fit, but didn't think they were too bad.

Since the levels of fitness did vary so much, some people found the early days of training so easy that it was some weeks before they felt any effect at all. Other people found Level 1 of both the aerobic and anaerobic training schedules totally exhausting. 'I think I was the only genuinely unfit person in my group,' said Fiona, a thirty-five-year-old school nurse. 'At the first session when we were meant to jog for five minutes, the others all went shooting off, but by the time I reached the sports club gates, I'd had it!'

As well as the medical tests, once the project was over all the participants were asked to fill in a detailed, thirteen-page questionnaire, prepared by GETTING IN SHAPE research fellow Hazel Belfield-Smith. The questions covered their feelings about health and fitness, their motives for getting involved in the project, their expectations of it, how it worked out in practice, and what they felt they had got out of it physically and psychologically.

Although obviously people's motives for joining the project varied, everyone said that the desire to improve their general health was either very important (79%) or fairly important (21%). 'I was attracted by the idea of discovering the minimum amount of exercise to keep ticking over,' one man said. 'This still is my main goal for the years ahead – far more important to me than becoming super-fit. At the end of the project, I would like to know how much fitter I am, and what is the minimum exercise I need to do in future to keep in reasonable shape.'

For four out of five participants, the specific aim of reducing the risk of heart disease was also a factor, though as you might expect, it was more important to men than to women. There were exceptions though. 'My father died of heart disease at fifty-eight,' said Joan, a civil servant in her late thirties, 'and his brothers had all died of the same thing before him. I know my father ate all the wrong things – lots of fried food – and though I avoid them, I have inherited his tendency to be overweight. When I read the *Sunday Times* article about GETTING IN SHAPE, I was thirty-seven and a half, feeling particularly fat and flabby, and thought that if I wanted to make it to forty, I'd better do something about it!'

Many people – two out of three, and men and women equally – hoped that they would lose weight as a result of exercise, and even more – almost three-quarters – hoped that it would improve their general appearance.

What appealed to many participants about GETTING IN SHAPE, as opposed to any other fitness regime, was that it offered a progressive exercise programme with specific goals under the supervision of trainers. Some were also attracted by the regular medical tests which they felt allowed them to push themselves harder than they would otherwise have done, safe in the knowledge that there were no problems with their hearts, lungs or blood pressure. A few were attracted by the idea of being part of a scientific experiment – being a 'medical guinea-pig' as one man put it.

Another element that seems to have attracted a lot of people to GETTING IN SHAPE is the fact that it was non-competitive. Indeed, many of them said they wouldn't have joined if it had been. Administrative director Will Chapman believes that dislike of competition stems basically from a lack of confidence, from the fear of looking foolish in front of other people. 'I suppose that among the non-athletic, this is often a hangover from the highly competitive nature of school sport. If you weren't athletic, you were a social outcast, and how many of us have experienced PE teachers who actually ridiculed those who weren't good at games?'

Claire, a journalist in her early forties, is among that number. Indeed, one of her reasons for choosing anaerobic exercise was that she thought it a good idea finally to try and conquer her fear of going into a gym. 'We were told that while aerobic training would improve stamina, anaerobic training would improve our strength and flexibility. That idea appealed to me very much. I like the idea of being able to stand my own ground, and deal with the awkward physical tasks that require precisely that strength and flexibility which most women don't have.'

The idea of exercising in a group attracted a lot of people – three out of four said it was an important factor. What appealed was the discipline that membership of any group imposes, which can be essential when self-discipline isn't that strong and the going gets tough; also, the kind of support that only fellow-sufferers can give, especially when they are from the same sort of background, have similar life styles and are just as embarrassed about the physical shape they are in!

Given the usual high drop-out rate in exercise projects the drop-out rate in GETTING IN SHAPE was surprisingly low. Around twenty-seven people – 15% – dropped out in the first six months, and around 25% in all had dropped out by the end of the year. It is hard to be precise about the figures because there is no foolproof method for defining drop-outs. Some of those who didn't return the questionnaire or attend the last session of tests may well have carried on exercising, while those who did return it or did attend the final session may well have stopped exercising. Some people were forced to drop out for reasons beyond their control – injury or illness, pregnancy, a change of job that involved moving house, or a change in family circumstances, a sick parent needing a lot of attention, for example.

Other people dropped out because they didn't enjoy it, didn't feel they were getting anything out of it, found that it was taking up too much time, or having missed a few sessions for reasons beyond their control, didn't feel sufficiently motivated to make up the lost ground.

Quite why the drop-out rate was so low, no one knows for certain, but one possible explanation is that many people found very quickly that they were getting a lot out of it. They enjoyed it, began to feel better within a few weeks, and if the second set of tests four months into the project confirmed a marked improvement in fitness they were strongly motivated to carry on. John, a solicitor of fifty who chose aerobic training, fell into that category. 'According to the second set of tests, I had reached the fitness level of an average twenty-year-old, and since I had really been feeling my age before I started, that was a terrific boost to my morale. I have a son of twenty who works as a gardener so he's pretty fit. When he took up running after I had, I was convinced that within a couple of weeks he'd be running right past me, but he isn't!'

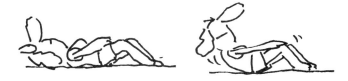

Many people were determined to finish what they had started as a matter of principle, and others – men more than women – were determined to avoid the sense of failure that dropping out would have given them. 'I actually told everyone I knew that I was doing the project,' said Joan, 'so that if I did drop out, the embarrassment would have been terrible, far worse than whatever it was that was causing me to waver! It worked, too. There were several occasions when I was seriously tempted to give up. I did find in the first six months that my legs hurt most of the time, and once the initial euphoria had worn off and I'd begun to think I'd always felt this good, that really did get to me and I thought about dropping out. The second time was when my group started to get very competitive about six months into the project. I was always at the back, and I hated it, especially when a couple of women in the group told me I wasn't trying hard enough! But the fear of facing all my friends and colleagues if I quit was enough to keep me going.'

Other people also considered dropping out, usually because they had been forced to miss a few sessions through illness or work commitments, but the group element and the commitment of the trainers were the factors that kept them going. Many people said they felt they would be letting down their colleagues and their trainer if they dropped out. A few disagreed. 'Although group motivation is important,' one woman said, 'individual motivation is paramount. You have to go through the pain for yourself. No matter how good the back-up and administration, you have to be prepared to do the pushing for yourself!' Other people who might have wavered felt a sense of responsibility to the project because it was a scientific study, and they believed that dropping out would have affected its validity, and on a more personal level, would have let down their unknown 'twin'.

Although it didn't emerge from the questionnaires, some trainers believe that competition with the unknown twin and curiosity about how well they were doing in comparison were important factors in keeping their members motivated, especially in the later stages of the project. It was for that reason, of course, that the GETTING IN SHAPE organisers did not reveal the twins' identities. The discovery that they had dropped out could have been very demoralising, as could the knowledge for some people that they were making much more rapid progress.

For one or two, the fact that they had invested £100 was a good reason to see it through, though perhaps the money was more important as a symbol of their commitment than anything else.

At the beginning of the project, the participants were deliberately not asked to change their diet, since the GETTING IN SHAPE physiologists were interested in how exercise alone affects weight. But they were asked to record any changes they did in fact make because the physiologists were also interested in how exercise affects eating habits. Just under half the participants found that their eating habits had changed during the course of the year. A few found they were eating more than before, and quite a lot of people found they had become more conscious of what they were eating.

'Becoming more aware of my body,' said Bill, a forty-three-year-old accountant, 'had led me to become more conscious of food and drink and its effects – positive and negative – on my system. I've cut down on booze and puddings because they interfered with the newer and better feeling of fitness. My diet and eating habits have improved, and I'm sure that's had an important effect not only on my health but on my state of fitness and the consequent, enhanced feeling of well-being.'

The majority didn't find that exercise altered their drinking habits, but of those who did most reported drinking less than before.

The participants were also deliberately not asked to stop smoking, but were asked to record any changes in their smoking habits during the course of the year. The vast majority – over four out of five – didn't smoke anyway. A quarter of them had smoked but had already given up before the project started. In some cases, that had been the first step in the decision to get in shape. Of the few who did still smoke, some cut down, seven carried on smoking as before and seven – more anaerobes than aerobes – gave up. Some of them found they no longer wanted to smoke, but for others it was a conscious decision. 'It seemed silly to be putting all this effort into getting fit,' said Claire, 'and at the same time continuing to fill my lungs with poison. The only problem I had with giving up was that I discovered I had a very sweet tooth, and so put on weight. But since exercise was turning a lot of the fat to muscle, that wasn't too high a price to pay.'

The physiologists were also interested in whether regular exercise affects sleep patterns, and if so, how. Although less than half the participants reported any change, for those who did, it was a real bonus.

'Although I'm a good sleeper,' said a thirty-seven-year-old occupational nurse, 'in times of stress, I used to wake feeling too alert in the mornings, and sometimes before the alarm. Now I feel the depth and quality of my sleep has improved, implying a greater degree of relaxation and relief of stress.'

David, a fifty-three-year-old marketing executive, feels his sleep pattern has changed too. 'Worries about work used to interfere with sleep before and keep me awake. But now, after a five-mile run, I fall into a very deep sleep. I wake five or six hours later – earlier than I used to – but that seems to be all the sleep my body needs these days.'

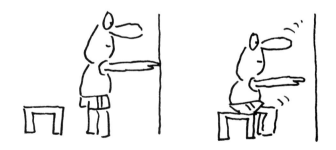

The questionnaires revealed very small differences in the responses of men and women, and in the majority of cases, between aerobes and anaerobes. But in one area, there was a marked difference – the enjoyment of the exercise programmes. When they were asked whether they had enjoyed the social side of the project, 82% of the aerobes said yes, while only 66% of the anaerobes said they had enjoyed it. Since the project set out to encourage the social element in every group by asking all the participants to get together for a drink after each weekly session, and in some cases aerobic and anaerobic groups met in the same place (though on different nights) and had the same trainers, perhaps the explanation for the differences lies in the nature of the two types of exercise. Jogging is a much more social activity than circuit training in a gym. Once you are over the initial breathless phase, it is relatively easy to jog in company and to chat as you run, whereas it is virtually impossible to do thirty-two rapid press-ups and hold a conversation at the same time, even if you are a world superstar. Quite a number of the aerobes arranged to run on their non-group nights with someone in the group who ran at roughly the same pace, whereas on their non-group nights, the anaerobes always exercised alone. Certainly the difference in the levels of enjoyment between the two groups is confirmed by the fact that while four out of five aerobes said they would be happy to carry on with the same type of exercise, over half the anaerobes said they would not!

The most common criticism of anaerobic training was that it was boring, especially in the latter stages when exercises were being repeated thirty or forty times in a session, and that it was very hard to see any progress. 'Okay, maybe I'd done two more press-ups than I'd done last time,' said one male anaerobe, 'but had I done them properly? At least with jogging, you know that if you've gone round the block a minute faster than you did the previous time, or if you've run half a mile further, you're getting better!'

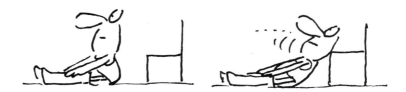

It was also much easier for the aerobes to set clear targets for themselves – the *Sunday Times* Fun Run, or possibly even a marathon – and work towards them. As one anaerobe put it, 'What's the equivalent for us? I can't see anyone organising a *Sunday Times* Fun Press-Up!'

Most of the discontented anaerobes said they would rather do aerobics, swimming, cycling or jogging, or possibly a mixture of aerobics and anaerobics. A number of anaerobes did in fact take up jogging once the year was over. Michael, a company director in his fifties, was one of them. 'I felt the seed had been sown and that I now had the chance to be the sort of person I'd always wanted to be physically. But I also felt that if I didn't carry on as soon as the project ended I would probably fall by the wayside. Since I'd felt from early on that the aerobes had been improving by leaps and bounds, I wanted some of that, and so I started running. The first time I went out was a severe jolt – even after a whole year's anaerobic training, I couldn't run more than 300 yards!'

Most participants planned to go on exercising once the project was finished, and in some cases, the GETTING IN SHAPE groups decided to carry on their weekly meetings once the year was up. About half of them felt they were doing enough exercise, although a third said they planned to do more.

'I'll continue with my weekly jog with the group,' one woman said, 'but I cannot *bear* doing it on my own, so I'll take up sprinting on the local track instead. I will probably do more sport generally, and never never again will I let myself get into the state I was in before I started!'

Although two out of three had said at the start of the project that they hoped to lose weight, only two out of five reported that they had done so. 'That was a disappointment,' said Joan, a civil servant in her late thirties, 'but then I didn't diet, and since I started GETTING IN SHAPE my weight has stayed the same. Up until then it had crept up every year, so without exercise I would probably be about a stone heavier than I am now.'

Two-thirds of the participants reported a change for the better in their physical appearance. Many women felt their overall shape was improved: arms, thighs and bottoms less flabby, stomachs flatter. 'I'm plump and muscular now,' said one female anaerobe, 'instead of plump and plump! I only wish that during the course of the year they'd taught us how to pose at bus stops so that it would be immediately obvious to everyone that here was a trained and toned body!' The men reported similar improvements: less flab, smaller waists and hips, disappearing beer guts.

Three-quarters of all participants found that their physical stamina had increased over the course of the year. People reported that they could get through their daily lives more easily than before, or that they were no longer limited in the things they could do by a lack of energy. Several people said they could now work in the garden all day without getting tired. 'Once I've got home from work and cooked a meal, I no longer feel that all I want to do is flop in a chair in front of the television for the rest of the evening.'

Perhaps the most interesting findings to emerge from the questionnaire concerned the psychological benefits that almost all the participants said they had experienced. Many people felt they had gained a greater degree of confidence and self-respect.

They felt more positive in their attitudes, more relaxed and less aggressive, and in a number of cases where a major birthday – forty or fifty – had been the cause of depression or anxiety, there was much less concern about the march of time.

'I feel that GETTING IN SHAPE has helped me come to terms with growing older,' said David, the marketing executive. 'I feel I'm much fitter now than I was in my thirties, or even my twenties, and that helps a lot. I must say I get a lot of secret satisfaction from knowing that under this grey business suit there is a good pair of legs that can comfortably carry me thirteen miles, which other people don't know about!'

Michael, the company director, admits to having been a very tense person. 'I was on tranquillisers for years, but I find now that I can run the stress out of me. I drive to Parliament Hill Fields, decide on a route and then abandon myself to the running. It's almost as if another person takes over – or at least another side of me. I wouldn't want to make extravagant claims for exercise, and it may well be just coincidence, but since I've taken it up, I'm enjoying life more than I have done for years.'

'It's actually made a great deal of difference to my self-confidence,' said Bill, a forty-year-old accountant who chose anaerobic training, 'and decisions are much easier to make and to stick by. I have an increased feeling of well-being, both mental and physical; I'm able to cope with the daily demands of work and home much better; and I have a reserve of energy left at the end of the day.'

'I feel much calmer than I used to be,' Clare said, 'and even friends have commented on it. I feel much more in control now, not just of my body but of my life. Things that used to restrict my activities just don't any more – like the fear of getting breathless and looking ridiculous, or the fact that it's snowing. Before, I would never go anywhere without being properly dressed and I had never ever worn a pair of jeans in my life. I used to spend a lot of time on my hair too, straightening it and making sure it looked neat. During the course of the year, I had it cut short and now I just towel it dry. It was very liberating!'

'Before, I really felt frail and fifty,' said a busy solicitor, 'tired and overstressed, but that isn't the case any more. Apart from losing masses of weight and feeling terrific, my mental approach to work is so much better now. It sounds Elysian, I know, but it's true!'

Jane, who's in her mid-thirties and has two young children, firmly believes that GETTING IN SHAPE is the best thing that has ever happened to her. When she started on it her marriage was breaking up and her confidence at an all-time low. 'I found it very hard at first just to motivate myself sufficiently to go along to the weekly session, and it was depressing always being at the back, but the trainers very quickly convinced me that it didn't matter. I could never have done it without the group though. The encouragement and the mutual support – and not just in terms of exercise – was absolutely tremendous.' By the end of the year, her self-confidence had not only returned but increased to the extent that she has applied for and got a place at college to do a psychology degree as a mature student.

Joan also feels she's changed as a result of GETTING IN SHAPE, though not necessarily for the better. 'I used to be much more patient than I am now. I didn't suffer fools gladly exactly, but I kept my feelings to myself. Now I'm much more likely to say what I think, and I don't think that intolerance is a good thing.'

Although many people who took part in GETTING IN SHAPE are very critical of some aspects of the organisation and administration, and to a lesser extent of the construction of the exercise programmes, there is no doubt that exercise itself, whether aerobic or anaerobic, has had a remarkable effect on their physical and psychological well-being. Certainly, the subjective findings – what the participants *feel* about exercise, their bodies,

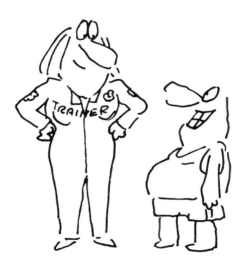

themselves and the resulting changes in their lives – were the outstanding feature of the project. 'Almost without exception,' said David Denison, 'the comments of the 104 participants who filled in the questionnaire at the end of the project were ecstatic. We really could not have hoped for a better testament to the benefits of exercise.'

Only one of the 104 participants who filled in the questionnaire claimed not to feel fitter at the end of the year, though as GETTING IN SHAPE research fellow Hazel Belfield-Smith points out, some people would be reluctant to say they felt no better after a year of exercise because they would be admitting by implication that perhaps they hadn't tried hard enough, and so that finding should be viewed with a degree of caution.

But she is greatly encouraged by the number of people who reported that being fitter has made it easier for them to cope with the physical and mental demands of their lives. 'Many people working in health education believe that this could be the key to convincing sedentary people who aren't currently motivated to exercise that it is a good idea. The message is not: take up jogging because you will be able to compete in lots of races or even run a marathon, and meet lots of interesting people. The message is: the physiological and psychological benefits that come from increasing your capacity to exercise, may help you cope more easily with your busy, demanding life!'

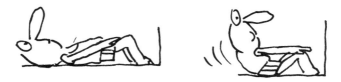

THE HOUSEWIFE AND MOTHER'S TALE

Diane, a lively, attractive woman in her late thirties, used to work with her husband in their graphic design business until six years ago when she gave up to have a family.

'I had three children in four and a half years so during that time I was either pregnant or just getting over being pregnant. I put on half a stone with the first two and a whole stone with the third, and weighing 10 stone 4 lb when I'm only 5'4" tall depressed me a lot. I knew I was eating too much and eating the wrong things, what with finishing up the children's food, or grabbing a bar of chocolate on the way to collect them from school if I hadn't had time for lunch. It was the possibility of losing weight that attracted me to GETTING IN SHAPE.'

Initially her husband wasn't keen. 'The baby was only eight months old, and he thought I was taking on too much, though once I'd started he was very enthusiastic. He'd come home early some nights to look after the children and sometimes he'd come and run with me.'

There were times early on when Diane herself wondered if she hadn't taken on too much. Going out for a run wasn't simply a question of putting on her trainers and going. It had to be planned like a military campaign.

'On my group night, for instance, the two elder children had their gym class, so I'd pick them up from school, bring them home, give them tea, take them to gym class, go and get the babysitter, bring her back here, then leave in time to get to my group, an hour's drive away, by seven. It would have been so much easier if I hadn't had the children, but then if I hadn't had them, I probably wouldn't have needed to do it!'

The children found it hard to adjust to the sudden change in their mother's way of life. 'The first few times I went out, the two elder ones stood by the window crying their eyes out. They had never been left before – either we took them with us or one of us would stay behind with them – and I suppose they thought I wasn't coming back! The babysitter said they'd stopped crying as soon as I was out of sight, and were fine, but it did make me feel awful!' Although it was difficult for her to get to the group sessions, Diane believes they were essential. 'If it hadn't been for the group I think I'd have given up. Most of the others were rather competitive and so I was too, and I felt that I had to keep up.' But Diane never found running alone a problem. On the contrary, she rather enjoyed it. 'In my life, I'm surrounded by people most of the time, so I quite looked forward to getting away from them all.'

For the first three months, her weight stayed more or less the same, much to her disappointment. But over the next three months, it started to fall off. 'I lost over a stone. It came off my arms, my waist and thighs, though not off my bust really, and even off my feet. Shoes that had pinched a bit before actually fitted comfortably. I went down a whole size in clothes, if not two. And I felt much fitter. My skin's got a glow that it didn't have before, and whereas I used to get the odd spot, I don't any more. I've been healthier too – running seems to act as a barrier to colds and other minor ailments.'

As the distances built up, Diane began to enjoy running and before the end of the project, she'd entered for the London Marathon. 'To me, it was a bit like taking the driving test. I'd started from scratch, had masses of help and encouragement from the trainers, and though the idea filled me with awe, running a marathon seemed to round the whole thing off.'

It was very hard going, finding the time to put in the necessary forty miles a week in training. 'I felt I was losing touch with the family to some degree, not seeing much of them, and when I did see them, my mind was on the next run and organising that. Towards the end, I almost resented the amount of time it was taking, but I knew I had to do it.'

She enjoyed the day, though never having run more than twenty-one miles before, she didn't know quite what to expect. 'I walked most of the last mile, though some of my group were manning the last water station in Northumberland Avenue, and I felt I really had to run past them. As soon as I was round the corner and out of sight though I stopped and walked!'

Now Diane runs between five and eight miles a week, and instead of running along the main road as she used to, she now runs through the local woods. 'What I want from my running has changed. Before, it was a competitive thing, timing myself over a measured distance, but now I go for the enjoyment of the countryside and the fresh air, rather like some people go for a drive in the country! I get home, have a shower, wash my hair and feel wonderful. A run is like a good night's sleep to me – I come back seeing things more clearly.'

Running has changed Diane's life. 'It's got me out of the house and encouraged me to make time in the day for myself. Once you are at home with children, it's very easy to give things up and do less and less for yourself.'

THE PUBLICAN'S TALE

'As far as health goes, running a pub is a pretty disastrous job, especially if you like beer as I do!' Nigel, who runs a pub in the City of London, stands 6'2" in his trainers, and weighs 18 stone.

'A few years ago I was managing a pub near Hyde Park and some of the members of the London Road Runners used to come in after their run for a drink. They used to try and get me to join them, but I didn't fancy it. I'm not really built for running! But they'd planted the germ of the idea of getting fit because when I read about GETTING IN SHAPE I wrote off straight away. I was very surprised to discover that a number of my former London Road Runner customers were involved in organising it, though I don't think I got any preferential treatment!'

Having discovered from the initial set of tests that being on his feet all day and heaving barrels of beer around had kept him fitter than he imagined, Nigel embarked on his anaerobic training programme with enthusiasm. 'I started to feel better almost immediately, though in a curious way it wasn't so much physical as psychological. I suppose the fact that I'd taken the plunge and was actually doing something about getting fit made me feel good.'

Given the hours publicans work, Nigel found it was a problem to fit in the three sessions he was meant to do at home every week. 'I don't finish much before midnight so obviously evenings were out and by the time the lunchtime session was over I didn't feel like doing it then either, so I used to get up an hour early, at 7 a.m., and do it then. It was never easy to kick myself out of bed, and the colder and darker the morning, the harder it was!'

Like most of his fellow anaerobes, Nigel found the routines pretty boring and occasionally relieved the monotony by cheating and going for a jog with the dog, but then he injured his knee and that put an end to that.

'I did have a week when I didn't feel too good at all, so I didn't exercise, and then I sneaked another week off too. But that only made it harder to get back into it because not only had I gone backwards, but the others had moved on a couple of levels. I'm very glad I did go back though and never seriously thought of dropping out. Once I'd committed myself, I could never have coped with the guilt!'

Nigel had hoped that he would lose weight, but he didn't lose more than a few pounds in the whole year. 'People said I looked thinner but I think what had happened is that some of the fat had turned to muscle and didn't wobble about so much! I didn't change my diet at all, or cut down on the beer. But then, one reason for exercising was to allow me to go on enjoying my beer with a clear conscience!'

The tests showed that his heart and lungs were working more efficiently at the end of the year, and he certainly felt better in himself. 'I'm very glad I did it because it's started me exercising. I've bought a bike and I now cycle the six or seven miles to work

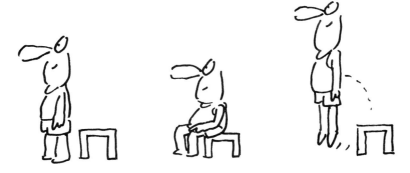

every day. The one real problem I had with anaerobic exercise was trying to fit it into a very hectic life, what with my job, my wife and children, and even the dog all wanting some of my time. Cycling to work is the ideal solution.'

THE HEADMISTRESS'S TALE

'I took my fortieth birthday very badly and felt I was going rapidly downhill. I was feeling particularly low about myself the day I saw the article about GETTING IN SHAPE and since the address to which you had to write was not far from where I live, I wrote the letter and dropped it off by hand that afternoon.'

Jane, a tall, attractive, lively woman, leads a very active, demanding life. She is headmistress of a school for emotionally disturbed children, as well as running a home and looking after a husband and three teenage children of her own. For the last fourteen years, she's been on drugs to control high blood pressure. 'When I approached my own doctor about taking part in the project, he said exercise would do me no good at all. But fortunately, the GETTING IN SHAPE doctors disagreed, and since the drugs I was taking were controlling the problem very well, they suggested I stayed on the same dose.' As Jane has never been able to run, she was happy to do anaerobic training. 'When I looked at Level 24 in the handbook they gave us, I thought I would never ever make it. In fact I was very pleasantly surprised at how quickly I made progress.'

The reaction of her family wasn't exactly supportive. 'My daughter went round saying, "My mum's a fitness freak. She is so boring!" My sons joked and jeered and kept saying I wouldn't keep it up. But then one day, they caught me doing sit-ups in the sitting-room and said, "How many of those can you do?" I replied casually, "Oh about thirty." So then they had to join in to show me how much better at it they were!

'The most resistance came from my husband in the form of silent resentment. He had been a keen tennis player but had to have a cartilage operation the previous year which had stopped him playing and he'd become very unfit. Having teenage sons telling him constantly how fat he was, and a sylph-like wife who suddenly had twice as much energy as he had rushing about the place, did cause friction.'

What kept her going in spite of all that and in spite of the long drive to her training centre every week after an exhausting day at school was a sense of commitment to the GETTING IN SHAPE experiment. 'I felt that if I dropped out I'd be letting down a lot of people, not least my "twin", whoever she may be. Actually finding the time to exercise wasn't a problem – you can always find time for something you really want to do – but motivating myself was. I never got into a routine and was always sitting in front of the television saying, "I'll go and do it in a minute!"'

Jane feels she reached her peak of fitness by the end of the first six months, although the *Sunday Times* Fun Run about that time which she'd been persuaded to enter, nearly killed her.

'I found I was full of energy and though I'm wary of claiming exercise as a universal panacea, I went through that year with hardly any of the migraines which I used to get quite often. Mine is a very stressful job and I used to have days when I felt I really couldn't cope. Now I feel exhausted at the end of the day but I never feel I can't cope. That is an unexpected bonus.

'As for my blood pressure, I decided a few months after the project ended to stop taking the drugs. I did feel pretty awful at first, but I expect that was withdrawal symptoms. After all, if you've been taking anything for fourteen years, your body's bound to react when you stop.

'I've lost over a stone in weight, and I've gone down at least one size in clothes, though I still find I instinctively take a size 14 off the rail and always have to go back and get a 12 or even a 10! I've got a much better body image than I've ever had and I even quite enjoy looking in the mirror now. Before our last summer holiday, I went out and bought the smallest bikini I've bought in years! I'd thought my bikini days were well and truly over, so that was very satisfying.'

Since GETTING IN SHAPE has ended, Jane has joined a local fitness centre and every week, in theory anyway, does one session in the gym, one aerobic dance class and goes out for a run. 'I still don't like running! Last summer a team of us from school – five staff and five children – trained for the *Sunday Times* Fun Run, and though I got round much more easily than I did the first time, it still wasn't easy!' She is also delighted that her husband, without any urging from her, has also enrolled at the fitness centre. 'It's taken him a long time to acknowledge what exercise has done for me, and to accept that it could do the same for him. I keep telling him that he'll have much more energy to do the garden, and the decorating, which may be a mistake!'

THE SOLICITOR'S TALE

It was John's wife, Sandra, a lively blonde in her late thirties, who spotted the original article in the *Sunday Times* and thought it would be a good idea for them both to apply. Not surprisingly, she was rather miffed when John was accepted and she wasn't. 'I knew they'd jump at a forty-year-old, overweight, stressed solicitor who said he was drinking too much,' she said good-humouredly, 'while I was obviously too ordinary! But I went along with John to the first meeting, and they agreed to accept partners who were keen to join in, which was terrific!'

John, a dark, rather quiet man, has his own legal practice in a north-London suburb, and found that the responsibility of being a one-man band weighed very heavily sometimes. So he had got into the habit of stopping off at his local pub on the way home for a few pints. It wasn't the effect of the alcohol that worried him so much as the calories. 'My weight had crept up to 13 stone 2 lb which is too much for someone 5'9½". I was forced to go out and buy new suits because I just couldn't get into the old ones any more, and slimfit shirts were definitely a thing of the past! Although I'd played football pretty regularly, I'd been saying for some time, "Tomorrow, I'll stop drinking, and start doing some exercise," but somehow tomorrow never came!'

During the initial testing before John started his anaerobic programme, his stint on the exercise bicycle showed that he performed much better and was much fitter than his way of life suggested he ought to be. 'It turns out that there is something in my metabolism which some highly trained endurance athletes have. The sports physiologists had always thought it was the result of hard training, but I appear to have it naturally, which got them very excited.'

At the beginning of the programme, John thought they were working at such a low level that the exercises couldn't possibly be doing him any good. And yet, from quite early on, he started feeling better. 'I stopped drinking as much. I made a conscious effort to stop popping into the pub on the way home, but I also found that when I'd been exercising I didn't want to drink anyway.'

He soon found the best time to fit in his three exercise sessions at home each week was in the lunch-hour. 'I work locally, so it was easy to come home, spend forty minutes doing my programme, shower, have a bite to eat and be back in the office within an hour and a half. I just couldn't have faced it in the mornings, and trying to fit it in after work would have been difficult.'

The biggest problem John had to deal with was boredom. 'For the first few months there was the novelty of it all. You could compare notes with the other members of the group but after that there really wasn't anything left to say.'

What kept him going was the support of the group, the fact that it was only for a year and the knowledge that it was doing him a lot of good. 'I found I really enjoyed the feeling of being fitter and the weight just seemed to drop off me. I lost two stone over the course of the year and all the new clothes I'd bought because I was putting on so much weight are no good at all to me now. I had expected to lose some weight, though not as much as I did, but what was a quite unexpected bonus was that I started sleeping much better and feeling much calmer about things generally. When I started I was feeling under a lot of pressure from work and not coping too well. I wasn't sleeping and so was very short-tempered. While I wouldn't claim I am now all sweetness and light, let's say that getting fit has lengthened the fuse!'

Once the end of GETTING IN SHAPE was in sight, John decided to set himself another target, because he felt that he'd probably slip back into the old ways if he didn't. He decided to start running and aimed at the Canterbury Marathon six months ahead. He aimed to do it in under three hours fifteen minutes, but finished in the very creditable time of three hours thirty-five.

'When we first started GETTING IN SHAPE, I did feel that I'd drawn the short straw in doing anaerobics. Certainly many people in my group did hanker after jogging and even did a bit, surreptitiously, though I wasn't among them. With hindsight, though, I'm glad I did it this way round because I was fit and strong before I started running. In the end I think we got the better end of the deal.'

Initially, he flung himself into his marathon training with too much enthusiasm. 'Sandra isn't competitive like me, and has a very sensible attitude to it all which stopped me from overdoing

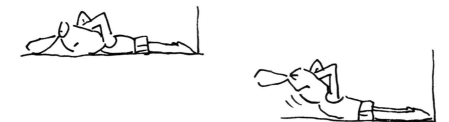

it. She'd say, "If you don't feel comfortable with the schedule, don't stick to it. Listen to your body." She was right – there is no point in forcing it.'

Looking back, John is in no doubt about the value of GETTING IN SHAPE for him. 'It was just the prod I needed to change the way I live, and I don't think I've got all the benefits from it yet that I'm going to get!'

THE WORKING MOTHER'S TALE

'I'd just turned forty and was very conscious of the fact that I'd put on weight because it was getting very uncomfortable to bend over while I was gardening. I was also aware that I was slowing down, so I felt I really needed to do something. When I read about GETTING IN SHAPE in the *Sunday Times*, I thought, "Fantastic!" and wrote off immediately.'

Hazel, a small, rather shy woman with bright eyes and a complexion like an eighteen-year-old's, works as a biology laboratory technician in a boys' public school. She has three children, all in their late teens, and a husband who's been a keen road runner for years. 'It wasn't realistic for me to start training with him because he was much too fast and besides, having

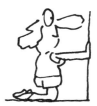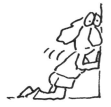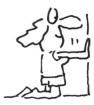

done no exercise for years, I was wary of just launching into it "cold". What appealed to me so much about GETTING IN SHAPE was the medical testing – not just because I'd know it was safe to start exercising, but because I'd have proof of how much fitter I had become.'

The first tests, before the project got underway, showed that Hazel's level of fitness was above average for her age, and the first aerobic training session with a gentle five-minute jog didn't cause her any problems at all. What she did find hard initially was jogging on her own. 'I felt really shy about going out alone, embarrassed that people might see me and think, "What on earth's a middle-aged woman like her doing running?" My husband came out with me a few times, but then, as a result of an article in the *Sunday Times* very early on, a woman who lived locally contacted me and we started running together once a week.'

As the distances she was covering increased, Hazel began to find it harder going. 'I was stiff for the first six months or so, and I lost weight only very gradually when I'd been expecting it to drop off me! If it hadn't been for the group, I think I would have dropped out during the early months. Certainly the fact that the others would know at the next session that I hadn't done the required amount of training during the week got me out on the road at times when otherwise I would have stayed put!'

As the amount of time involved increased, Hazel found it harder to fit the training into an already very busy life, what with a full-time job and a family to look after. Other interests had to go – sewing, knitting, evening classes in cookery and even a half-completed Open University course.

However, by the time she injured a hamstring six months after the project started, running was an essential part of her life. 'I went to see my doctor who said I'd have to give up running for good. The physiotherapist I saw said, "I'll only treat you if you stop. I don't like runners!" I did as I was told for a couple of weeks, but I missed the running so much that I gradually started again. When I spoke to a sports physiotherapist at the West London Institute, he told me I'd done the right thing – the sort of injury I had needed some exercise to push blood through the muscle.'

Nine months after GETTING IN SHAPE started, along with some other members of her group, Hazel entered the Paris— Versailles 10-kilometre race, and found to her surprise that she was more competitive than she'd ever imagined. She entered for the London Marathon the following spring, and finished in a very creditable time of just over four hours. 'I loved it! It was so exciting with all the people along the route cheering for you. It's as though they sense when you're beginning to flag and call out your number urging you on.'

Looking back at GETTING IN SHAPE, Hazel feels it's changed her in lots of ways. 'I lost 10 lb and the tests showed that I had much less body fat than before. Certainly my shape has changed. But, more important, I feel so much younger now and so full of energy. I'm also much more self-confident than I used to be. As a direct result, I've now started a running club for women locally, and I really enjoy helping other women to start running. I think we have many more psychological barriers to overcome than men. They don't mind people seeing them red-faced and sweaty, whereas many women still do!'

It has changed her home life too. She now understands and shares her husband's pleasure in running, and her children have had to become more independent. 'I certainly don't rush round after them like I used to – I just don't have the time – and I'm sure that's done them good. And housework is now very firmly at the bottom of my list of priorities!'

Hazel's immediate goal is to get under four hours in her next marathon, and she simply can't imagine her life without running now. 'My only regret is that I didn't take it up twenty years ago. Then I really might have got somewhere!'

THE CARTOONIST'S TALE

'I blame school. They put tremendous emphasis on being good at games and I just wasn't. I'd be forced to do the cross-country and even when I cheated and took a short cut, I still came in last! As a result of all that, from the second I left school I did nothing physical at all and since I eat junk food and drink quite a bit – up to two bottles of wine a day – I hit forty-five horrendously unfit.'

Gray, a cartoonist and advertising copywriter, is a large, striking-looking man with a shock of untidy grey curls. Having read endless newspaper articles about health, he was worried about the state of his own, and had even taken the first, tentative steps towards doing something about it.

'I asked my doctor if I should take up jogging and he said, "At your age it would be like holding a loaded gun to your head!" Certainly I was aware of people I knew dropping dead after they'd suddenly taken up exercise. So I found myself on the horns of a dilemma – being told by the media that I'd drop dead if I didn't take exercise and being told I'd drop dead if I did! The GETTING IN SHAPE project came along and that seemed to offer the chance to do it under the supervision of people who weren't going to let me do anything super-strenuous.'

Given his memories of running, it's not surprising that he opted for anaerobic training, but found to his dismay that even that involved a small amount of running – once round the outside of the gym.

'I could feel my heart pounding and I was convinced I was going to die. I was thinking, "I don't want to go this way. I want to die overeating!" And afterwards, I always got a terrible headache – much worse than any hangover I've ever had.

'The other thing I have against running is that London air is absolute filth and there you are sucking down great lungfuls of it! I did toy with the idea of designing a mask – a bag with holes for your eyes and a silly face painted on it that would actually filter the air that you breathed. It would also be very good for people who were embarrassed to be seen out jogging by people they knew!

'One other thing about the project that didn't make sense to me was that when we'd finished exercising and, hopefully, working off some weight, we'd retire to the local pub, drink several pints of beer, and put it all back on again!'

About nine months into the project, Gray had a particularly nasty bout of flu and missed three weekly sessions. 'When I did go back the others had progressed quite a lot. The following week, I found some excuse not to go, and that, basically, was that.

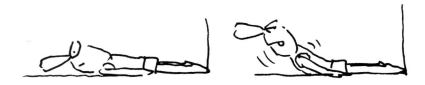

'All the time I was exercising, I didn't lose any weight and I didn't change shape. There may have been some stomach muscles developing, but they never made it to the surface through the layers of fat. I still look like a rope with a knot in the middle! I can honestly say that I never felt better for a minute. In fact once I started I found I kept getting ill, which I'd never been before. The trainer said it was a sign that I was getting fitter, but it didn't make sense to me that I had to feel ill and terrible in order to get fit! Perhaps I just didn't push myself hard enough. I never even reached the pain barrier, never mind went through it. But then I'm not very keen on pain, I'm a hedonist, not a masochist, and that was the problem. I have nothing but praise for the scheme and for the trainers – the fault was all mine. Self-discipline has never been a very strong suit.'

But the guilt hasn't gone away and he still worries about being unfit. 'Every time I get a twinge in my chest, I say, "This is it! I should have kept going." It's not that I don't have any will power at all. I have. I gave up smoking just like that but then I didn't have to go anywhere to do it. Perhaps if I could have been beamed up and put in the gym, ready changed, then beamed home again, changed back and showered I'd have been more successful!'

THE DOCTOR'S WIFE'S TALE

Jean, a small, plump, energetic woman has always led a very full, active life what with bringing up her teenage daughters, helping her husband who's a GP run his weekly gynaecological and obstetric clinic (she trained as a nurse and midwife) and pursuing her hobbies of mineralogy and jewellery making. But fifty loomed and she felt the onset of middle-aged spread very keenly indeed. Her main aim in joining GETTING IN SHAPE was to lose some weight and since, as she says, she wasn't built for running, she opted for anaerobics instead. The first session confirmed that she really needed the exercise.

'It was so undemanding really, and yet I came away feeling weak and trembly, as though I'd really been working hard!'

Although she was only meant to exercise on alternate days, Jean decided to exercise every day because she felt that if there was a gap, she might be tempted to stop altogether.

'Within three months, I really felt the benefit. I've suffered from backache most of my life – it's a minor congenital problem – and more recently from neckache too, but they both went. I felt much livelier, bouncier, and I didn't tire as easily as I had before. We go skiing every year, and on the previous holiday, I'd tired quite easily and the rest of the family overtook me. This time, when the rest of my class got tired, I didn't. I could have gone on all day!'

During the course of the year, Jean discovered a hidden talent. 'At the Sports Day we had at the West London Institute, no one from our group would volunteer for the short sprint, so I did. I've always run on my toes, and the race nearly killed me. My calf muscles were agony! But then our trainer recommended the right running shoes, taught me how to run properly and I discovered I was really quite fast! One day at our training centre, the secretary of some athletics club who'd seen me do a couple of 60-yard dashes asked me if I'd like to join his club because they were short of women sprinters! I didn't take him up on it, but I was very flattered!'

With her medical background Jean took the tests very much in her stride, although, like many of her colleagues, she hated the bicycle at the West London Institute with a passion. 'In the test before we started training I only managed six minutes, and I was determined to improve. But at four months and eight months, I still only managed six minutes. It became a real object of loathing and I was determined that it wasn't going to get the better of me. I even enrolled at a local gym so that I could get in some practice on an exercise bicycle. On my final test I managed eight minutes.'

But Jean already knew that she was much fitter by the end of the year than she had been at the start. 'On the first day I found it impossible even to do the full number of wall push-aways (kneeling in front of a wall, hands on it and arms straight, bending your arms till your nose touched the wall and then pushing away). By the end, I could do thirty proper press-ups!'

Her one major disappointment was that she didn't lose any weight. 'Nor did I change shape. I know that a lot of the fat had turned to muscle, because the caliper tests showed that the percentage of body fat had gone down, but it would have been nice if it had showed!'

For Jean the group element was vitally important. 'I really enjoyed the company and made some good friends. If you're all sweating and suffering together you can't help but get close!'

Before the end of the project, Jean had enrolled at a local gym and carried on going for a while after GETTING IN SHAPE had ended. Then she joined the rump of the aerobics group at the same centre, and carried on until that finally petered out. 'Now I try and do something every day – run or swim or, if I can't get out, then I'll do some exercises at home. But I know that I'm not as fit as I was – I can't do thirty press-ups anymore – and that's a shame. I think I'm the sort of person who needs the incentive of a group to keep me going!'

THE MERCHANT BANKER AND THE EXPECTANT MOTHER'S TALE

Over the years, David, a large jovial chap of forty, and his wife Sandra, a slim, attractive woman who's three years younger, have had their fair share of injuries. In his mid-thirties David smashed a couple of vertebrae, and Sandra had a serious road accident a few years ago and broke both her legs. Although she had played basketball to national standard in her younger days, by the time her legs had mended, any vestige of her former

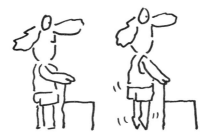

fitness had vanished. Her major motive for joining GETTING IN SHAPE, though, was to try and give up smoking, while David's was to lose weight, since any excess poundage aggravates his back injury, causing him more or less constant pain. His work involves him in a great deal of social eating and drinking, so dieting wasn't a realistic option, and that, combined with the fact that his job is pretty high-powered and stressful, made him an ideal candidate for exercise.

Although he says he was very unfit when he started GETTING IN SHAPE he didn't find the early sessions of aerobic training too difficult. 'I hurt a bit after the first few runs, but after that I was aware that my body was working better, and within about five months of starting I ran a half-marathon. Once your heart, lungs and leg muscles are strong enough, then it's all in the mind!'

Two months later, just over seven months into the project, a friend who had a place in the New York Marathon had to drop out, and although the race was only a matter of weeks away, David took up the challenge. He trained hard, even running to and from his office in the City to make sure he got the mileage in, much to the amusement of his colleagues.

'About two weeks before we flew off to New York, I was out running one evening, and I felt my body really run free for the first, and I'm sad to say only time. It was a glimpse of paradise and I got close to understanding why athletes are athletes. It was certainly the highlight of the year for me.'

He finished the New York Marathon in five hours, though he is now convinced that cramming the training into such a short space of time was a mistake and certainly would not recommend it to anyone else.

'Afterwards, I was ravenous, and I didn't stop eating for about three months. I'd managed to get my weight down to about fourteen stone during the project, but then it started to creep back up again, and now, what with being too busy to run and doing a lot of entertaining, I'm back to around 15½ stone. But at least I know that if I put my mind to it, I can take it off again without too much trouble.'

Sandra, who has two children aged eleven and nine from a previous marriage, found that she started to feel better soon after she began exercising, but instead of it making her want to stop smoking, it made her feel less guilty about carrying on!

About two months into the project, Sandra discovered she was pregnant. 'I told the GETTING IN SHAPE doctors about it, but they said there was no reason why I shouldn't carry on. In a way, being pregnant helped me see the project through, because I was determined that it wasn't going to interfere with my life at all!'

She never grew particularly large, and the bump didn't interfere with her running. 'The problem was my boobs – trying to run with all that extra weight up there and not knowing quite what to do with them!'

Eight months pregnant, she took part in the *Sunday Times* Fun Run, and finished in a very respectable time. 'But I did stop running a week or so after that because I was frightened I might fall and damage the baby and it just didn't seem worth taking that chance.'

Sandra is convinced that being fit made the delivery easier and David, who was there, agrees. 'We were both extremely good at the panting!' A few weeks after the baby was born Sandra tried to start running again, but she felt she'd fallen a long way behind the rest of the group, and besides, broken nights and exhausting days sapped her energy.

'I carried on to the end of the year because I felt I ought to, but my heart wasn't really in it. Once GETTING IN SHAPE had finished I was able to say out loud what I'd gradually come to realise – that I *hate* running, that it's boring, and I really can't see the point!' She laughed. 'I took great delight in telling the rest of my group so, too! I still go along to the group nights and thoroughly enjoy myself, but that's all. Although the tests showed that I was fitter at the end of the year, to be honest I don't really feel any different!'

THE TAXI DRIVER'S TALE

'When I passed joggers in the street I used to admire their bottle. Now when I see them I say a prayer!'

Dominic, a thirty-eight-year-old East-ender, drives a cab in central London and divides the blame for the stressful nature of his job between the traffic and the members of the public he picks up. Whether they were the direct cause or not he doesn't know, but about the time GETTING IN SHAPE was announced he found that he was suffering from high blood pressure.

'My brother saw the article and pointed it out to me, thinking it might help bring my blood pressure down. I'd already given up smoking in the hope that might help, but all that had happened was that I'd put on weight. I hoped that the project might help me lose it.'

The first set of tests showed that his blood pressure wasn't as high as it had been, but before he could actually start on his programme of aerobic exercise he had to have his tonsils out. 'I started a bit behind the rest and it took me a long time to reach the top level – Level 14.'

He had more than his fair share of illness during the year. A few months in, he picked up chicken pox from his six-year-old son and was in bed for three weeks. 'That was the closest I came to giving up the whole project. It was very hard to get back into it again. It didn't bother me that I was so far behind the others – they'd always been better than me anyway – and in fact it was the group, and the trainers that got me going again. They could see I was struggling and really gave me a lot of encouragement – kept telling me that I was one of their success stories because I kept at it, even though I found it so hard!'

For Dominic, running never became easy, and it was always an effort to go out on his own. 'I'd come in tired and hungry about six. You can't run on a full stomach so unless I went there and then, before my supper, it meant waiting until nine or ten o'clock, and of course I was nicely settled in the armchair by then. But I did make myself go out most nights. I felt I'd be letting the others down if I didn't!'

His wife was all in favour of the project and always encouraged him to go out. 'I took a lot of ribbing from the bloke next door. "It's bad for you, all that jogging!" and that sort of thing. And to start with I did feel very self-conscious setting off down the road in my running-gear. But I got used to it eventually.'

Dominic didn't lose the weight he'd hoped to lose, nor did he begin to feel noticeably better, so for him the four sets of medical tests were very important: the only guide he had to the progress he was making. 'After the second set of tests they showed me my chart. My lungs were pretty good to start with so there wasn't much progress there, but my heart was working much more efficiently, which was very reassuring.'

Looking back, Dominic doesn't really know what he got out of the project. 'From a physical point of view, I can run further than I could before, and I must admit that running does help me unwind at the end of the day. Now that the project's over I still go training with a group one night a week, and I try to run at least once a week with a mate. It's much better running with someone and chatting to take your mind off what you're doing than running by yourself. But it is still an effort. I still have to force myself, and I can imagine all too easily not running. I suppose what keeps me going is the knowledge that it's doing me good, even if I don't feel it!'

THE CLERGYMAN'S TALE

'In the mid-seventies I worked in Bangladesh and came back very healthy and thin, a mere 10½ stone. But then I was appointed chaplain of a Cambridge college, and five years of high-table living with too much good food and drink on offer meant that in spite of fairly regular games of squash I put on over two stone. My doctor told me my blood pressure was up and that the best thing I could do was lose some weight, so any fitness programme that was disciplined and organised would have caught my eye. Being fit – like avoiding sin – is a Good Idea!'

Bob, who's forty-one and currently working at Church House, the administrative headquarters of the Church of England, opted for aerobic training but said he would accept either, and was in fact put into an anaerobic group. 'I was glad to be accepted at all, though initially I was a little disappointed at how slowly we progressed. I had expected to suffer a bit more! But after the first six weeks I began to feel I had made progress and at the second set of tests, four months in, there was very clear evidence that I was fitter, which was encouraging.'

Bob's present job involves a lot of travelling to conferences all over the country so it was never easy to find a regular time to do his three solo exercise sessions. 'It didn't help that the routine itself was deeply boring, but you just had to grin and bear it. Besides, the corporate element – not wanting to let the group down and the knowledge that you would be tested so that any backsliding would be evident – was a very strong incentive to keep going! I also made a point of telling lots of people that I was in the GETTING IN SHAPE project – insurance, if you like, that I would see it through!'

About halfway through the year, Bob and some of his fellow anaerobes were asked by the GETTING IN SHAPE organisers to take part in the *Sunday Times* Fun Run, just to see whether their anaerobic training had improved their aerobic capacity at all.

'I was very conscious that the few short runs we'd done had left me more breathless than I should have been and since the Fun Run is 2½ miles I did go into training for it. I worked quite hard but I didn't do anything like as well as I'd hoped. It was a real set-back to be honest, and I found it much tougher immediately afterwards to keep going. But I was never seriously tempted to give up – the original motivation stayed with me and I really enjoyed the group sessions, especially the drink afterwards!'

The highlight of the year for Bob came during the third set of tests on the bicycle at the West London Institute. 'I was able to keep going for three minutes longer than the previous time and the doctors told me that I was in the top 10% of people my age in the general population. That was very rewarding.'

By the end of the year Bob hadn't lost the weight he'd hoped to lose – 'The thin man inside me is still trying to get out,' – but he knows that he is much fitter. 'At the moment I'm renovating an old house, and I know the amount of physical labour I've been doing would have exhausted me a year ago. Now it's not a problem.'

When the year was up Bob's group were asked if they'd like to carry on with pure anaerobics, switch to pure aerobics, or to a mixture of the two. Bob gratefully accepted the mixture – some warm-up exercises, a run, followed by a session in the gym with weights. 'If I'd been told eighteen months ago that I'd be running 6 miles without it being a tremendous effort, I simply wouldn't have believed it. I suppose I could imagine giving up exercising, but I can't imagine ever giving up sport. Being fitter has certainly enabled me to enjoy sport more. I play squash more often and don't get anything like as tired as I used to.'

THE HEALTH EDUCATION OFFICER'S TALE

As a former PE teacher and now a health education officer in south London, Margaret was very well placed to judge just how unfit she had become. 'Over the years I'd gradually given up all the sports I used to take part in, and though my husband is a keen tennis player I finally let that slip too. The GETTING IN SHAPE project struck me as a real chance to get fit again, and since I can usually do things if I'm egged on, I applied.'

At the first session of her anaerobic group, Margaret felt rather embarrassed at being seen in public in a tracksuit. 'We had to jog on the spot for one minute – it felt like ten! – and I was frightened to look round in case anyone was looking at me! The one problem I had initially was that as we exercised as a group I couldn't go at my own pace. I felt silly if I was still swinging my arms when the others had finished and were waiting for me to move on to the next exercise.'

After a couple of months, though, there was no doubt that Margaret was feeling fitter and stronger. 'I had an overgrown allotment to sort out and I found I could manage a day's heavy clearing and digging without feeling tired. I didn't lose any weight, though. They did tell us at the start that we wouldn't necessarily, but I'd thought that if I ate sensibly I would.'

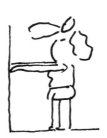 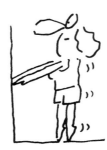

Margaret's job is very demanding and she's also active in several organisations in her spare time, so after four months she found that various committee meetings had forced her to miss several group sessions in succession.

'The next week I decided I'd do my exercises at home and then go and join the group for a drink afterwards. For one thing it was very hot and I preferred exercising in my underwear at home. I preferred the privacy, too. I even hated it if one of my daughters came into the bedroom while I was exercising.'

That soon became the pattern. Margaret would exercise at home and then join the group for a drink. 'I suppose if I'm honest I never really got anything out of exercising in a group, but I really did feel the exercises themselves were doing me good. I had bags of energy and once again experienced the pleasure of feeling bright and bustling and just plain fit – something I hadn't felt for years. My hips were slimmer too, my body was firmer, and my face looked fit – people were always telling me how well I looked! I even started jogging a bit as part of my warm-up, until I injured myself running on a beach on holiday in France.'

When she did go back to a group session in September, after the summer-holiday period, she found only three other people there. 'I suppose that was the beginning of the end. I did keep on exercising by myself, started jogging again, and though I was putting on weight, I did feel I was still getting fitter.

'By Christmas, though, I'd stopped, and my training diary for January and February records a few feeble attempts at exercise with comments like: "I am so *unfit*; *all* my own fault." Now I'm not doing anything at all.'

But while Margaret accepts that it's partly her own fault, she does feel that the project let her down rather badly. 'I'm angry that in my group anyway no attempt was made to chase up the drop-outs. I understand it was policy not to do so because the motivation to keep going was one of the things the scientists were looking at. But we had made a contract with them. We paid £100, we were going to help them and they were going to help us get fit. I think if someone had rung me up and said they'd noticed I had missed a few sessions it would probably have pricked my conscience and I may well have carried on.

'I also resented the fact that after the first few sessions no one bothered to look at our training diaries. I kept mine religiously, even if I missed the sessions, and I never cheated, but what was the point when no one saw it! In health education we talk a lot about the "contract" between the "professionals" and their "clients" who want to diet or stop smoking or drinking, to help them through the sticky patches. That's what I needed and that's what I didn't get.'

THE TRAINERS' TALE

Patrick and Brenda, trainers of the North London aerobics group, are both in their mid-fifties, though they look ten years younger and have the energy and enthusiasm of people half their age. But while they have all the missionary zeal of true converts, it's tempered by great good humour, and the still vivid memory of what it's like to be middle-aged and unfit.

Although they both now have administrative office jobs, Brenda trained as a dancer, appearing in West-End shows at night and attending classes every day, which kept her in such good shape that she was a finalist in the Miss Great Britain contest for four years running. When she and Pat married in 1953 she gave it all up. 'I did some modelling, but when our son was born I stayed at home, put on a lot of weight – about 2 stone – and became a fat, jolly lady! I didn't think I minded too much, but one day my agent rang up and offered me some outsize modelling, and that really hurt! I did try all sorts of diets at home but none of them worked, and I just wallowed in my fat for years.'

Then, about ten years ago, she heard about Weight Watchers. She joined, and within seven weeks was down to her target weight. Although she was looking better she didn't feel any better, largely because she was still smoking about forty cigarettes a day. 'And then we had a huge row about it because I'd gone through 800 duty-free cigarettes in a couple of weeks. A few days later, I said I was going to give up, and I stopped just like that. The first three weeks were murder, what with physical withdrawal symptoms, but I survived.'

Once the withdrawal symptoms had gone she began to feel better and looked around for some gentle form of exercise. 'I took up yoga because I liked the graceful movements, and it

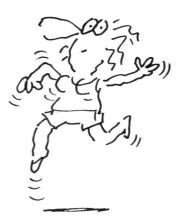

wasn't competitive. After a year I was asked if I'd like to train as a teacher and I qualified three years later. It was very useful training as things have turned out because we learnt about physiology, about the structure of the body and how it all works.'

Pat was delighted that Brenda had taken up a physical activity because he had always played football and cricket at weekends – 'Badly, but I enjoyed it!' – and was interested in all sport. That's why he went along to watch the first London Marathon in 1981. 'I stood outside Buckingham Palace in the pouring rain and waited until the last oldies had finished. I was so impressed by the spirit of the runners and by the sheer endeavour that I went home, put on my trainers, and ran down the road and back. I decided then and there that I'd train by myself for the '82 Marathon and not tell a soul except Brenda that I was doing it! People think that because I'd played football and cricket regularly I was fit, and therefore it was easy for me. It wasn't, though – that sort of exercise is quite different.'

Shortly before the '82 Marathon Brenda read about the 'Fun Runner '82' project, and having seen what running was doing for Pat she applied to join without telling him. 'I knew he'd make fun of me if I told him, so the first he knew was when the trainer rang to say that I'd been accepted and to warn me how tough it was going to be!'

At the party given for the runners the night before the London Marathon Pat discovered that the prime movers in 'Fun Runner '82' were members of the 82/50 group – people like himself who'd decided to run their first marathon, but who'd trained together.

'They still ran every Saturday morning in Hyde Park and after the '82 Marathon changed their name to the Serpentine Running Club. We joined and that really changed our lives. They were so welcoming, so supportive and so understanding of middle-aged people wanting to get fit.'

When GETTING IN SHAPE was launched Pat and Brenda were invited to become trainers. 'We were delighted to be asked, though we felt we were really only beginners ourselves. But then Brenda's yoga training had given her a good grounding in physiology, and we thought that since we were oldies ourselves we wouldn't let our people do anything rash or silly, so we decided to give it a try!'

Their main objective was to train the members of their group to run and to stay free of injury. 'In fact we had no injuries at all in our group. If people were becoming too competitive, or trying to rush things, we tried to hold them back without dampening their enthusiasm.'

In the early days some of the group members were disappointed that they weren't losing weight. 'I'd tell them to forget about the scales and concentrate on the tape measure,' said Brenda. 'Since I've been running I haven't lost a lot of weight but my bust has gone from 38 B to 34 C. What's happened is that most of the fat's come off my back! I also tell them that today's look is healthy, trained and toned for men and women, and that's what exercise gives you.'

Their group was one of the most successful. Not only was the drop-out rate during the year very low, but at the time of writing, a year after the project ended, a large number of the members still attend the weekly group session.

'I think the key to motivating people was always to find ways of doing things as a group, so we'd always start together and then come back together again before the end of the session. The social thing is very important, and so we always made sure that people had someone to run with. For the vast majority of people the "Loneliness of the Long Distance Runner" is not what it's all about!'

They both got enormous satisfaction from seeing people transformed physically and psychologically during the year. 'Of course it's exciting to see people who've done no exercise for years running a marathon. But it's just as rewarding to see the look of joy on the face of someone who had thought of the

Sunday Times Fun Run as a bit like climbing Everest, after they've just done it!'

Brenda ran her first marathon at the age of fifty-four in 1983, and in 1984 she and Pat ran four marathons, including London and New York. Exercise is their life now. Brenda teaches yoga and dance aerobics three nights a week; Pat plays squash at least twice weekly; on Thursdays there's the group that grew out of GETTING IN SHAPE; on Saturdays they always run with the Serpentine Running Club in Hyde Park; and most weekends they compete in a race somewhere.

Although they enjoy all their sporting activities they both agree they can't imagine their lives without running now. 'When I see old ladies walking along all bent over,' said Brenda, 'I just can't imagine ever being like that. Of course I'll get older, but I can't see myself being old. It really has changed my life. I feel great, I look better and my self-confidence has improved a lot – I'm quite cocky now.'

3

EXERCISE AND YOUR BODY

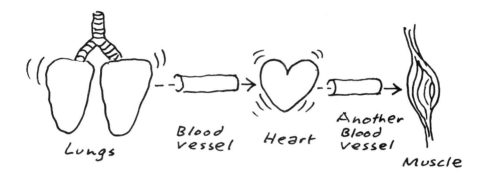

Lungs   Blood vessel   Heart   Another Blood vessel   Muscle

HOW IT WORKS

Even the simplest action you carry out involves many of the body's intricate, interrelated systems working in unison. Lifting a finger, for instance, involves not just the muscles, bones, joints and skin, but to some extent the nervous system, the endocrine system, the heart, lungs, circulation of the blood, liver, kidneys . . .

As far as exercise is concerned, though, the most important systems are the cardiovascular system – heart, lungs and circulation – and the muscles. The heart, made largely of cardiac muscle, is essentially a pump designed to push blood around the body by means of arteries, veins and the smaller arterioles and capillaries – some 60,000 miles of blood vessels altogether.

Each time your heart beats it pumps oxygen-rich blood out of the left ventricle (one of the heart's four chambers) through the body's tissues. At rest, the brain gets about 25%, the other organs like the liver, and systems like the reproductive system get 55% between them, and the muscles, although they make up around 40% of body weight, only get around 20%. The moment you start to exercise, the distribution of blood flow becomes very different, because the oxygen delivered to the muscles by the bloodstream is essential for the production of energy which they need in order to work. At the same time the bloodstream removes the waste products created in the process – heat, water, carbon dioxide (CO_2), and lactic acid.

The heart speeds up, pumping blood around the body faster, and almost all the extra flow goes to the muscles. The flow to other parts of the body remains largely unchanged. However, as you begin to get hot, you need the extra blood to radiate away the heat that's been generated from the skin. (Incidentally, 80% of the energy produced by the body is wasted as heat. Only 20% goes in useful work.)

The water that is made by the muscles is eventually passed out through the bladder as urine or as sweat through the skin.

Carbon dioxide is transported by the bloodstream through the veins back into the right atrium of the heart and then, via the right ventricle, into the lungs where it is exchanged for oxygen.

As you breathe, air passes from the bronchi (larger airways) into the broncheoli (smaller airways) and finally into the alveoli (air sacs). No one knows precisely how many alveoli there are, but estimates vary between 300,000,000 and twice that number! On the surface of each alveolus is a network of capillaries, and as molecules of carbon dioxide diffuse from the blood through the walls of the alveoli to be breathed out eventually, so molecules of oxygen pass in the opposite direction, from the alveoli into the haemoglobin in the red blood cells. (It is the oxygen that gives haemoglobin its red colour.) It's estimated that the total surface area in the lung, where the exchange of oxygen and carbon dioxide takes place, is approximately the same as a tennis court! The oxygen-rich blood is then pumped back from the lungs into the left atrium, then into the left ventricle, and the whole cycle starts all over again.

Muscle accounts for 40% of our body weight and there are three different types – smooth or involuntary, cardiac, and skeletal or voluntary. Smooth muscle works automatically in the digestive, circulatory, urogenital and respiratory systems. Cardiac muscle, as its name suggests, makes up most of the heart and is special in that all its cells contract and relax in the same rhythm. Skeletal muscle holds the skeleton upright and enables it to move around.

Both cardiac and skeletal muscle deteriorate if they are not worked hard. They lose both strength and bulk, and they shrink. Many people become less muscular as they grow older, but this is the result of under-use, not an automatic consequence of old age. Fortunately, skeletal muscles respond rapidly to exercise. No matter how long it is since they worked hard, and no matter how weak they have become, the process is not irreversible and after a few weeks' exercise, they will increase in bulk and strength. (Incidentally, women have fewer muscle fibres than men, so their potential for muscle development is less, and a woman who takes regular exercise won't automatically wind up looking like a body-builder.)

There are two types of muscle cells – white or 'fast twitch' and red or 'slow twitch'. The former are used for short, sudden bursts of activity and work anaerobically – without oxygen. The latter are used in endurance activity because they have a high capacity for taking up oxygen in myoglobin – the muscular equivalent of haemoglobin – which gives these particular muscle cells their red colour.

All muscles need fuel in order to work, and the fuels stored in the body for this purpose are glucose, which is immediately available but lasts only a few hours, and fat which takes longer to mobilise but which lasts much longer – several days.

Glucose comes from the carbohydrate in our diet and is stored as glycogen (chains of glucose molecules) in the muscles themselves, and in the liver. Under normal circumstances, most people have about 9 lb of glycogen stored in their body.

Fat, or adipose tissue, is stored all over the body. In women it is under the skin, distributed evenly all over the body, which is why women are more curvaceous and have a higher percentage of body fat than men. In males, on the other hand, body fat tends to be stored around the abdominal organs, which is why they get a paunch if they are overweight and women don't. Fat is used as fuel by the muscles in two forms. It can be broken down into Free Fatty Acids, or it can be converted into glycerol and then into glucose.

Glucose is converted into energy by a complex biochemical process. Basically, what happens is that muscle cells absorb glucose and in the mitochondria (the hundreds of minute cellular powerhouses that each cell contains) the glucose molecules start to break down, step by step, into a substance called pyruvic acid. In the process, small amounts of energy are produced and are trapped by a compound called Adenosine Di-Phosphate (ADP), uniting with a third phosphate to form Adenosine Tri-Phosphate (ATP), the common currency of energy in the body. The stored energy is released when the third phosphate is split off again, and the compound reverts to being ADP. In fact it is that process which triggers the breakdown of the glucose molecules in the first place.

What happens once the glucose has been broken down into pyruvic acid depends on whether or not there is oxygen present. If there is, then the pyruvic acid is broken down by a cycle of enzymes in the mitochondria (called 'Kreb's Cycle') into water and carbon dioxide, releasing large amounts of energy in the process. The energy is then trapped by ATP, which in turn gives it to the muscle to work. The process is called aerobic glycolysis. A small amount of the oxygen needed for this process is stored in the muscle's myoglobin – enough for about ten seconds' running – but most of the oxygen required is provided by the haemoglobin carried by the bloodstream.

If there is no oxygen present then the pyruvic acid breaks down into lactic acid. When there is a build-up of lactic acid, all energy-producing activity in the cells ceases, and the muscle feels tired, or even cramped. Anaerobic glycolysis, as it's called, is a very effective way of producing instant energy in a very short period – to allow you to run for a bus, for example. It produces energy five times faster than aerobic glycolysis, but it is a very wasteful process because it produces only about 5% of the energy that aerobic glycolysis would produce from the same amount of glucose, wasting a lot of it as heat, and only producing small amounts of ATP.

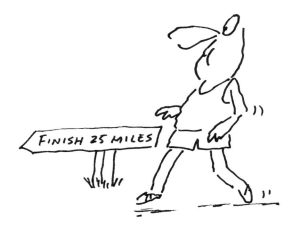

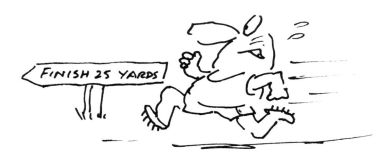

If you think of ATP as the body's energy currency then in aerobic exercise you are only spending it as fast as you produce it. In anaerobic exercise, though, you are going into debt as your body can't continue to manufacture the energy you need fast enough. After you finish exercising, that debt has to be repaid. That's why you go on breathing hard and why your heart goes on racing after you've stopped exercising, so that the anaerobic reserves can be replenished.

Under normal circumstances, when the muscles are working aerobically, both water and carbon dioxide are produced. The water is carried to the bladder and the carbon dioxide is transported by the bloodstream back to the lungs where it is exchanged for oxygen.

One of the most important functions of carbon dioxide in the body is the regulation of breathing by controlling the breathing centres (groups of cells) in the brain. If you over-breathe and flush out too much carbon dioxide, your brain tries to protect itself from the loss by shutting down its blood vessels. It does it so effectively that it also cuts off its own oxygen supply so that you lose consciousness. This allows the brain to resume total control of your breathing, restoring the carbon dioxide in the blood to an acceptable level and opening up the blood vessels again so that you regain consciousness.

All these processes take place while you are at rest, or just ticking over. When you exert yourself, though, the body responds in a remarkable way. The speed at which the blood circulates round the body increases by up to *six* times. Working flat out, the heart can pump 40 pints (23 litres) of blood round the body in one minute and deliver about 1 gallon of oxygen. The volume of blood flowing through the working muscles increases by up to *three* times. Some of the blood that would have gone to the digestive or reproductive systems is diverted to the muscles. Since the blood is also circulating six times faster, that means there is an *eighteen*-fold increase in the total amount of blood reaching the muscles.

As the muscles start to work harder they produce more carbon dioxide which stimulates the breathing centres in the brain so that you start to breathe faster. The number of breaths you take doubles, and the amount of air you take in each time increases so that the total volume of air inhaled is up to *twenty* times greater. Since the muscles are demanding more oxygen to do the increased work, a network of small capillaries opens up within them, bringing the blood into closer contact with the muscle cells so that more oxygen can be extracted from it. The amount of oxygen extracted by the working muscles increases a staggering *fifty-four*-fold. At rest, the muscles only extract about 25% of the oxygen available in the blood, but working flat out they extract up to 75%. That three-fold increase, multiplied by the eighteen-fold increase in the blood supply, results in that fifty-four-fold increase.

Since the blood is now flowing through additional channels, your blood pressure drops and the heart responds by pumping faster to bring it up to an acceptable level again. And, of course, the fact that the blood is being pumped back faster to the heart by the working muscles also speeds up its output. If it didn't, there would be a build-up of returning blood in the veins waiting to be pumped through the lungs, re-oxygenated and pumped out again.

If the heart is normal and healthy the extra blood flowing into it at a slightly increased pressure stretches the muscle more than usual. As a result it contracts more strongly and pumps out more blood. Your systolic blood pressure – the pressure when your heart is actually pumping the blood out – will rise to cope with the added demand from your muscles. The diastolic pressure – the pressure between heart beats – will remain more or less the same.

As for fuel, the harder the muscles work, the more they will need. When you start to make more demands on them they respond by first using their own stored supply of glycogen and then drawing on the stores in the liver – a total of about 9 lb. During sustained activity (anything longer than twenty minutes) the body will start to call on its reserves of fat. Several hormones, including adrenaline, are released to help break down adipose tissue into Free Fatty Acids. They are then transported to the muscles where substances found in glucose are needed to start the chain reaction which leads to the production of ATP and, therefore, energy. (The reason why endurance athletes sometimes break down is not that their stores of fat are exhausted; it's that none of the enzymes needed to start that chain reaction are left.)

When you stop exerting yourself and have something to eat carbohydrates are first converted into glucose for immediate use, and then into glycogen to replenish the stores in the muscles and liver. Unless you eat more than you need for those purposes the body fat that has been used up will not be replaced.

The rate at which the rest of your body uses up fuel – your Basic Metabolic Rate – can be increased during sustained activity by up to 30%. Research done in Norway a few years ago showed that the Rate was still around 10% higher twenty-four hours after activity had ceased.

If you exert yourself regularly – take exercise, in other words – a number of long-term changes, beneficial to your health and sense of well-being, take place in the body, depending on the type of exercise you do.

It seems clear that the amount of exercise you can do is limited primarily by two factors – how fast your cardiovascular system can deliver oxygen to your muscles, and how effectively your muscles can extract that oxygen. To some extent, these factors are genetically determined. No matter how hard or for how long they train, most people will never be able to run faster than a six-minute mile simply because they were not born with the necessary equipment. But there is no doubt that for most people regular exercise can improve the efficiency of their cardiovascular system. Like skeletal muscle, cardiac muscle responds to exercise – working harder than usual – by becoming bigger and stronger. As a result, each contraction of the heart is stronger and therefore each stroke pumps out a greater volume of oxygen-rich blood than before. Since the heart now needs fewer strokes to pump out the same volume of blood it is working less hard and is therefore under less strain. That means that as you get fitter, not only does your heart rate rise much less during exercise than it did before, but you can carry out your ordinary day-to-day activities with less strain on your heart. And, like any piece of machinery, the less hard it has to work to achieve the same result the longer it should last.

The major direct effect of training of any kind, though, is on the muscles. In anaerobic training – weight lifting, circuit training, sprinting and so on – where white or 'fast-twitch' muscle cells are used, the body produces more white cells which give the muscles greater strength. It also produces more of the enzymes which are essential for anaerobic glycolysis – the production of energy without oxygen.

While this kind of exercise will have no effect on the 'slow-twitch' or red muscle cells, aerobic training will increase the production of enzymes for producing energy in both types of muscle cell. The mitochondria, the cellular powerhouses, respond to aerobic training by increasing in number, and the amount of myoglobin – the red muscle cells which take up oxygen – increases from 2% of muscle weight to 5%, providing a cushion against the need to draw on your anaerobic reserves. The number of blood-carrying capillaries in the muscle also increases with regular exercise – from around 600 per square millimetre to around 850 – which means more oxygen is available to your muscle cells for energy production and your stamina is increased.

Since your muscles have become more efficient at extracting oxygen from the blood flowing through them, it means that under normal circumstances they need less blood to supply the required amount of oxygen and so the heart doesn't have to work so hard in pumping it round the system. Again, the overall result is that you use less energy in carrying out your daily tasks and so you feel less tired.

As we said earlier, when you exert yourself the rate at which the rest of your body burns up fuel is increased by up to 30% and twenty-four hours later it can still be up to 10% higher. By exercising regularly – every other day ideally – for a minimum of twenty minutes, it's possible to raise your metabolic rate permanently by up to 15%, so that even when you are at rest or asleep your body is burning fuel at a faster rate than before. The effect is maintained as long as you exercise regularly. One reason why this happens is that you are developing more muscle and muscle burns fat as fuel. Many people feel rather disappointed when they start exercising regularly that they don't lose weight, but the fact is that many of them will have lost body fat and gained muscle, which is heavier than fat although it takes up less space. Initially, a tape measure is probably a better guide to progress than the bathroom scales.

Incidentally, if you try to lose weight by dieting alone your body will eventually lose both fat and muscle, and since there will be less muscle than before to burn up fat you will need even less food to meet your body's needs and you could find yourself trapped in a downward spiral. In addition, your body interprets the sudden drop in food supply as a crisis and so your Basic Metabolic Rate slows down in order to preserve what resources there are, so it becomes harder and harder to lose weight.

THE TESTS

All the participants in GETTING IN SHAPE went through four sets of medical tests at the Brompton Hospital in South Kensington and at the West London Institute of Higher Education in Isleworth. The first tests were done before they started training, and then at four months, eight months, and twelve months when the project finished, to see what progress, if any, they had made.

First of all, they were weighed and measured, and the percentage of body fat was calculated. To do that, the technicians test a pinch of flesh using specially calibrated calipers from four different places – the back of the upper arm, directly over the shoulder blade, the top of the hip bone and the abdomen. The four figures are then added together and a calculation done which produces a figure for the percentage of body fat. In this project, under 15% was considered good, between 15% and 30% overweight, between 30% and 45% badly overweight and between 45% and 60% very seriously overweight.

Although the medical team did not expect all the participants to lose weight during the course of the year, tests done previously on people during a training programme showed that their shapes changed as a result, and one very effective method of monitoring that change is optical contour mapping done by the 'stripey light' test. Two equidistant projectors project a pattern of narrow vertical stripes against a blank wall. The participants – men stripped to the waist, women wearing shorts and bandeau-style bikini top – stood against the wall, their hands above their head, holding on to a bar. The distortion of the stripes caused by the contour of their bodies was then photographed three times. The first time, they were asked to take as deep a breath as possible and hold it. The second time, they were asked to breath out normally, and the third time, to breathe out as far as they possibly could.

The 'stripey light' test can be used to calculate the volume of the torso and changes in volume, but it is an extremely time-consuming process. As far as GETTING IN SHAPE participants were concerned, the simple visual comparison of previous 'stripey light' photographs with the current photographs showed very clearly if weight had been lost, from where, and how the body shape had changed.

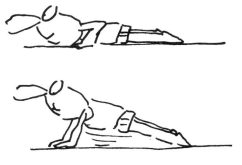

The participants also underwent a series of lung-function tests at the Brompton Hospital. The first was the Maximal Flow-Volume Loop Test – or Floop Test for short – which shows if the lungs are working normally, and if they are not offers clues as to what the problem might be. The equipment, in crude terms, consists of a mouthpiece leading into a bellows inside a box attached to a computer which measures the amount of air breathed in and out – the 'Volume' – and the rate at which it is breathed – the 'Flow'. With a clip on their noses to ensure that they breathed only through their mouths, the participants were asked to take as deep a breath as they could before the test actually started. Then they were told to breathe out as hard and as fast as they could until their lungs felt empty and then to breathe in again, also as hard and as fast as they could.

By comparing the trace produced by their Floop Test with a trace that can be predicted according to age, height and sex, it was easy to see whether their lungs were working normally, and to spot any problem like asthma, bronchitis or emphysema.

The second lung-function test was Whole Body Plethysmography or the 'Body Box'. The object of this test was to find out how large the participants' lungs were, and to measure the resistance of the lungs' airways. The subjects sat inside an airtight box, breathing through a mouthpiece attached to a pressure gauge. There was another pressure gauge attached to the box itself to measure the pressure inside it. As they breathed out against the first pressure gauge, the amount of air in their lungs was squashed, the space it occupied reduced and so the pressure rose. Since the air then took up less space in the lungs, the amount of space around them inside the box increased, and therefore the pressure dropped. From the rise in pressure measured by the mouthpiece gauge and the fall in pressure measured by the box gauge, the volume of air in the lungs, and

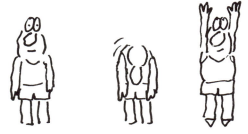

therefore their size, could be calculated and compared with the expected size, predicted from age, height and sex. Lungs bigger than predicted are usually the result of obstructed airways or weakening of the alveoli, the minute air sacs at the ends of the broncheoli. Lungs that are smaller than predicted usually result from a stiffening of the alveoli. This test also showed the level of resistance in the lungs' airways. If it was higher than predicted, it indicated obstruction in the airways, possibly as a result of asthma, bronchitis or emphysema.

The third lung-function test was the Gas Transfer Test which measures the efficiency of the lungs at transferring oxygen into the bloodstream and removing carbon dioxide from it. The equipment – basically a mouthpiece linked to a supply of oxygen-rich air mixed with minute quantities of helium and carbon monoxide – is linked to a bag which collects the air breathed out and a computer which analyses it. With their noses clipped, the participants were told to empty their lungs, then breathe in as much of the mixture as possible and hold it for ten seconds.

Helium is insoluble in blood and so cannot escape from the lungs. But it can be diluted by gases already in the lungs, so by analysing how much weaker the concentration of helium has become the computer can calculate the Accessible Gas Volume (VA): the amount of gas in the lungs that could be reached by the helium in ten seconds. Carbon monoxide (CO), unlike helium, is very soluble in blood, so the amount that is removed during the ten seconds it is in the lungs is a measure of the volume of blood reached by the VA in that time. Both the VA and TLCO – Transfer by Lung of Carbon Monoxide – can be predicted according to age, height and sex, and comparatively high or low values on the test can indicate damage to the blood vessels in the lungs.

As well as the lung-function tests, all the participants underwent heart examinations at the Brompton Hospital.

Echocardiography uses sound waves, rather like an echo-sounder on a ship, to build up a very accurate picture of the heart, its shape, size, thickness of walls, working of valves, and relative timing of the movement of the various parts. It is done by holding the sounding device against the chest. It picks up the echoes and translates them into a picture on a screen.

The participants also underwent electrocardiography – ECG – which makes use of the fact that the heart generates a small pulse of electricity to start each beat. By placing a number of electrodes at various points on the body – inside the wrists, on the leg, on the chest and back – the course of this electrical impulse can be plotted with great accuracy, and any abnormalities of rhythm, strength and distribution can be spotted very easily. After a coronary, for instance, an area of the heart muscle is destroyed to the extent that it can no longer conduct electricity, so it's easy to see from the shape of the trace whether someone has suffered a heart attack in the past.

All the tests at the Brompton Hospital were carried out while the participants were 'at rest', but at the West London Institute they were carried out during exercise.

The testing was done on an ergometer – a fixed exercise bicycle – rather than on a treadmill because on the former it's much easier to measure exactly the amount of work done. On a treadmill, as he runs, one person might jump twice as high as another person, and therefore do twice as much work, even though the amount of time spent and the 'distance' run would be the same for each. On a bicycle everyone spends almost the same amount of energy to push the pedals round at the same rate.

Before the test started, the participants had a blood-pressure cuff wrapped round their left arm, a series of electrodes stuck on their chest and back and wired up to the computer. Their left earlobes were pricked so technicians could take samples of arterial blood (oxygen-rich blood on its way from the heart) at intervals throughout the test – painful, though nowhere near as painful as having an artery slit. With a clip on their noses, they were asked to breathe in and out through a mouthpiece. They breathed moisturised air to prevent their throats becoming dry during the test.

They were told to start cycling at a pace sufficient to keep the needle on the dial fixed to the handle-bars at a set reading, and to keep going until they felt they couldn't carry on, either because their legs gave out or because they were out of breath. As they cycled the work load was increased by 25 watts every two minutes so that they had to pedal harder to keep the needle steady. 30 microlitres of blood were taken from their earlobes every four minutes and examined for levels of blood gases and for lactic acid. The increase in their heart rates as they exercised was monitored closely, as were the rate of breathing and the size of each breath, and the composition of the exhaled air was examined for oxygen and carbon dioxide. When they stopped pedalling they remained wired up for a further minute so that their recovery rate (an important indicator of fitness) could also be monitored.

Since everyone needs the same amount of oxygen to do the same amount of work, what the results of the bicycle test show is how hard the heart has to work to pump the oxygen required by the muscles to do the work – in other words, how efficient it is – and also how efficiently the lungs pump out carbon dioxide.

The blood tests show how much oxygen the lungs are able to transfer into the blood, and how the amount varies as exercise progresses. The levels of lactic acid indicate the point at which the muscles become deprived of oxygen because lactic acid is produced when the muscles are working anaerobically – without oxygen.

The results of the same tests repeated at four, eight and twelve months, would show clearly what effect training had on the efficiency of the cardiovascular system.

THE RESULTS

GETTING IN SHAPE presented the physiological team from the Brompton Hospital and the West London Institute with a unique and exciting opportunity to collect data on a large number of normal, averagely healthy people. Although they were not a random cross-section – they had, after all, selected themselves by responding to the original article in the *Sunday Times* and were, by definition, concerned about their state of fitness – they were close enough to the normal population to be of great value to the team.

Since most exercise testing in the past has been done on athletes, physical education students or people suffering from disease, the team wanted to check before they actually started on GETTING IN SHAPE that the 'normal values' used in the standard tests were likely to be applicable in this instance. The standard predictions used for lung-function tests, for example, are based on groups of people from different geographical, social and occupational backgrounds, and are therefore all slightly different. So, as a preliminary trial, fifty-one visitors to the lung-function laboratory at the Brompton, whose ages ranged from eighteen to seventy-two and who had no recent history of either heart or lung disease, were recruited and subjected to lung-function tests.

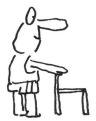 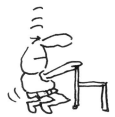

It was found that the most commonly used prediction under-estimated the '1-second Forced Expired Volume' or FEV1 (the amount of air that can be forced out of the lungs in one second) by 7%, the 'Forced Vital Capacity' or FVC (the amount of air that can be taken in in one deep breath) by 10%, and the Total Lung Capacity or TLC by 5%. On the other hand, it overestimated the Whole Lung Carbon Monoxide Transfer or TLCO (the amount of carbon monoxide absorbed by blood vessels in the lungs: an indication of the volume of blood available in the lungs to absorb oxygen) by 4%. Since the GETTING IN SHAPE participants came from similar backgrounds to those in this pilot study, the team expected to find similar deviations.

It found another small but significant deviation in a much smaller pilot lung-function study. It found that the Accessible Gas Volume was only approximately 87% of the predicted Total Lung Capacity.

In the same way, the team also carried out preliminary tests to check on 'normal values' for progressive exercise tests, both on cycle ergometers and on motor-driven treadmills, on two groups of healthy but sedentary people. The results varied so little from the predicted norm that they were not considered statistically significant.

The GETTING IN SHAPE participants turned up for the first

round of testing at the Brompton Hospital and the West London Institute before they embarked on their chosen exercise programmes.

The lung-function tests showed that the group was normal and their results consistent with what the team expected from the pilot study of fifty-one people. They also showed the effects of smoking on lung function. Only twenty-two of the GETTING IN SHAPE participants smoked, and only thirteen smoked more than ten cigarettes a day, but their results showed clearly the expected effects of smoking. Their Forced Expired Volume (FEV1), Forced Vital Capacity (FVC), Unforced Vital Capacity (VC – the amount of air normally taken in in one breath), Transfer in Lung of Carbon Monoxide (TLCO), and volume of blood per litre of lung (KCO) were all below those of the rest of the group, indicating damage to the small airways which was denying incoming gas access to various parts of the lung. Their Total Lung Capacity (TLC) and Residual Volume (RV) – the amount of air left in the lungs, when you have breathed o ıt as far as you can – were raised, however, and the amount of gas remaining trapped in their lungs (TLC minus VA) was greater, resulting from damage to the small airways which made the lungs larger.

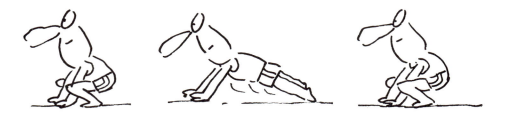

When the lung-function results of the aerobes and the anaerobes were compared after the first series of tests they showed that the TLC and the TLCO of the anaerobes were on average 3% and 5% less respectively than the aerobes, which means that not only were their lungs slightly smaller but they also had less blood in them and so they were slightly less fit.

From the answers given in the questionnaire, David Denison concludes that the difference was due to self-selection. 'Many of the anaerobes opted for that form of training for negative reasons – they didn't want to run, perhaps because they didn't think they were fit enough to.'

The first exercise tests were designed to measure aerobic capacity, maximum heart rate and ventilation rate against both aerobic capacity and carbon dioxide output. The wide range of general fitness levels among the GETTING IN SHAPE participants at the start was obvious from the length of time they managed to keep going on the cycle ergometer before either their lungs or their legs gave out. Some people, both men and women, had to stop after only two minutes, while one man, a solicitor of fifty, kept going for fifteen minutes! Since it was expected that many people would not be able to keep going long enough to demonstrate a true aerobic capacity during the first test, the physiological team decided to estimate it from their peak oxygen consumption (Vo_2 Max), which is sufficiently closely related to aerobic capacity to provide a useful result.

The initial tests showed that on the whole the GETTING IN SHAPE participants were slightly overweight and sedentary but normally healthy people. As expected, the aerobes did better on aerobic capacity: the women achieved 99.4% of what was predicted according to sex, age and height, and the men 99.8%; the anaerobes achieved 91.2% and 89.7% respectively. Again, David Denison believes this to be a reflection of their choice of exercise programme rather than anything else.

Four months later, at the second round of testing, 154 people turned up. 145 turned up for the third round of tests eight months into the project, and 119 turned up for the last set of tests at the end of the twelve months. Since most of the physiological changes had taken place by the end of eight months, the team chose to concentrate on the 145 people who turned up for the third round of tests.

AEROBIC CAPACITY

The female aerobes showed a 15% increase in aerobic capacity, which they had partly achieved by the end of four months and fully achieved by the end of eight months. The male aerobes showed a similar but slightly smaller increase. As you might expect, the anaerobes showed much less of an increase in aerobic capacity, since their training was not designed with that in mind. The women showed an increase of 8.5% by the end of the eighth month, though that had fallen back to around 5% by the end of the project, while the men showed an increase of 5% by the end of the eighth month, though that had almost disappeared by the end of the year, leaving them more or less where they had started. This falling-away could well be due to the fact that a number of anaerobes found it very difficult to keep motivated once they had reached the end of their exercise

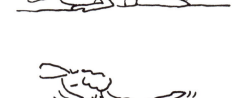

programme and the peak of their fitness – the idea of increasing the number of circuits or the number of exercises within each circuit, the only options open to them, wasn't very appealing – and, therefore, found it harder to keep on exercising.

HEART RATE

The expected effect of training on the heart rate is that it will decrease as the heart becomes stronger and more efficient, and therefore needs to work less hard to achieve the same result. On the cycle ergometer some people were so unfit at the first test that their leg muscles became too tired to carry on pedalling long before their heart had reached its maximum training rate, and so at subsequent tests, their heart rate had increased. For instance, Serena, a thirty-two-year-old teacher who opted for aerobic training, only managed two minutes on the bicycle during the first test, with a maximum heart rate of 159 beats a minute. At the third test, though, she managed to keep going on the cycle for eight minutes and her maximum heart rate was 185. The following April, she managed a very respectable time in the London Marathon! At her first exercise test, Betty, a fifty-one-year-old housewife, managed four minutes on the cycle, with a maximum heart rate of 193. At the end of the year she kept going for twice as long and her heart rate was down to 185 at double the work load.

The female aerobes on average showed a reduction of 10 beats a minute and a 14% increase in maximum work load which was largely achieved by the end of the fourth month, fully achieved by the end of the eighth month and that improvement was sustained until the end of the year.

The male aerobes showed an even more marked improvement. Here, the average reduction in heart rate was 20 beats a minute, clear at low work loads by the end of four months and at all loads by the end of the eighth month. At the first test, the maximum heart rate of David, a fifty-year-old executive, was

180, but twelve months later it was down to 160 at double the previous work load – a very significant improvement.

The female anaerobes showed no significant changes in heart rate throughout the year, while for the men there was at most a reduction of 4–5 beats a minute at low work loads only.

LUNG-FUNCTION TESTS

Again, most of the improvements in lung function took place in the first four months of the project. The aerobes (both men and women) showed small but statistically significant changes. The Forced Expired Volume showed an improvement of 2%, Forced Vital Capacity also 2%, unforced Vital Capacity 1.4%, and Volume Accessible 3.3%. These figures indicate a significant improvement in the mechanics of the bronchial tree, most probably in the small airways, which would result in people feeling less breathless, although a more efficient cardiovascular system delivering more oxygen to the muscles and muscles producing less lactic acid would also play a part here.

The anaerobes showed an even more marked improvement in lung function, especially in the measurements where they had fallen behind the aerobes in the first test. Total Lung Capacity (TLC) increased by 2%, as did Whole Lung Transfer of Carbon Monoxide (TLCO), and the Accessible Gas Volume (VA) increased by 4.2%.

The third set of tests – at eight months – showed that the improvements made by both groups had been kept up and even increased, especially in Accessible Gas Volume, while the anaerobes continued to show a definite increase in TLC and TLCO. In fact, by the end of the year, the anaerobes had more or less caught up with their aerobic partners. According to David Denison, what these results suggest is that training improved members of the two groups according to their needs. 'The anaerobes had more potential for improvement in lung function than the aerobes so that's the effect the training had. Although I can't prove it, I suspect that there would have been the same improvement in lung function if this group had done aerobic exercise.'

There is no doubt that the men and women who took part in GETTING IN SHAPE were in better shape at the end of the twelve months than they had been at the start. The one exception perhaps is the woman whose results in the exercise tests remained exactly the same on all four occasions. The likeliest explanation is that she just didn't train enough, if at all, because the effects of even a small amount of training would have shown up as an increase in the litres of oxygen per minute she consumed, even if her time on the cycle and her maximum heart rate had remained the same.

As for one of the main purposes of the project – to compare the relative merits of aerobic and anaerobic exercise – David Denison is reluctant to draw too many conclusions. 'There's no doubt that aerobic training is more fun and much less boring than anaerobic training, and that is a good reason for choosing it. But in other ways the choice depends on what you're setting out to achieve. It's foolish to try and improve your tennis by practising the piano! If your aim is to improve your aerobic capacity, then not surprisingly, aerobic training is more effective than anaerobic training.'

Whether or not aerobic capacity is the best indicator of physical fitness and well-being is another matter. David Denison thinks on balance that it is not. 'Certainly the benefits gained by participants in GETTING IN SHAPE are out of all proportion to the improvement in aerobic capacity.

'I think aerobic capacity should be abandoned as a yardstick for anything except laboratory tests, because it is not closely related to real life. For most of us, life is at least a sixteen-hour event every day, with at least eight hours continuously on the go, and it may be that stamina which is not measurable at the moment is a better guide to fitness.'

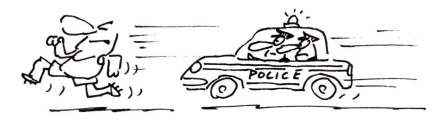

4
PUTTING IT INTO PRACTICE

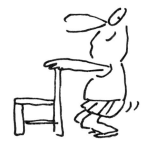

One thing that GETTING IN SHAPE showed conclusively is that it is perfectly possible for any middle-aged, sedentary, overweight, reasonably healthy but unfit person to get in shape on approximately two hours' exercise a week in eight months or less, without causing any unwanted major upheavals in their day-to-day lives. So if you fall into that category and want to get in shape yourself, how should you go about it?

The results of GETTING IN SHAPE seem to have borne out a theory that Malcolm Emery of the West London Institute has had for some time – that most people who start exercising after many years of inactivity actually need to get in shape for getting in shape. They often find that their heart and lungs are in better condition than their muscles, so if they start jogging, say, they'll find that their leg muscles are so tired that they have to stop long before their heart reaches its training level – the rate it needs to reach before it will start getting stronger and working more efficiently.

'You also find that when people are unfit, not only are their muscles getting weaker through lack of use, but their weight is going up, so when they start to jog there is additional strain on their calf muscles particularly. During GETTING IN SHAPE, that showed up as soreness and sometimes injury. There were quite a few people in the aerobics group who were in pain for several months. Ideally, what they should have done was a few weeks' swimming or cycling, where their body weight would have been supported, or some initial anaerobic exercise to improve the condition of their muscles before they started jogging. And not simply for strength either. It's pointless training the heart to deliver more oxygen to the muscles if the muscles haven't the capacity to extract and use it. Exercising and strengthening the muscles encourages them to open up an infrastructure of small capillaries so that more blood passes through them and more oxygen can be extracted.

'Certainly, some of the people who did anaerobic training for a year and then started running found it much easier than they would have done if they had started "cold" because they were already fit and strong and their muscles were able to use the increased oxygen that their cardiovascular system was delivering.'

Malcolm Emery believes that most people can get fit enough to start getting in shape in about twelve weeks, though obviously it varies. 'We found during GETTING IN SHAPE that people who had once been fit could regain a reasonable level of fitness more quickly than people who had never been fit.'

As the results of GETTING IN SHAPE showed very clearly, the two different types of exercise resulted in improvements in different areas – aerobics in more efficient heart and lung function, and anaerobics in better lung function and also in greater flexibility and muscle strength. So for people whose heart, lungs and muscles are all in much the same state, perhaps the ideal exercise prescription initially is a mixture of the two. Three twenty-minute sessions of aerobics – jogging, swimming or cycling – and one session of anaerobics, either simple exercises or weight training to improve muscle strength and tone. A programme like that once a week for four to six months should be enough to get most people in shape. As the results of GETTING IN SHAPE showed, the improvement in the heart rate of most participants was largely achieved by the end of the first four months, and fully achieved by the end of eight. The same was true, by and large, for aerobic capacity.

Once you are in shape, Malcolm Emery believes that two half-hour exercise sessions a week ought to be enough to keep you in shape. 'Most people don't want to be super-fit. They want to be able to enjoy life to the maximum with the minimum amount of effort, and they want to be reassured that they are pretty healthy.'

Most of the GETTING IN SHAPE trainers felt that six months was long enough to establish the habit of regular exercise. Anyone who hadn't got the habit by then was very unlikely to, no matter how much longer the project went on.

Another valuable lesson learnt from GETTING IN SHAPE is that people need an exercise programme geared closely to their present level of fitness, and also to their expectations. 'It's pointless starting someone who's really not that unfit at the lowest level – not only is it a waste of time, but they are likely to lose interest – and it's equally pointless pushing someone who has not the slightest interest in running a marathon into running further and faster all the time. For that reason, the development of fitness centres is a good idea. People can go in and have their level of fitness checked out, and then on the basis of that information they can decide what they need and what sort of exercise to do.'

It also emerged very clearly from the participants' answers to the GETTING IN SHAPE questionnaire that for the majority of people the group element is extremely important. As one man put it, 'It's extremely easy to start exercising by yourself – and extremely easy to stop!' So how do you go about finding a group? Many towns now have a health club or gym with all the latest equipment, but they do tend to be expensive and you may find that most of the other people there are first-class specimens of the Body Beautiful brigade, admiring their rippling muscles in the mirrored walls, which can be extremely off-putting if you are overweight and out of condition yourself. It is very important to find a group of people in roughly the same state of fitness as yourself, which means asking at your local sports centre or adult education institute for beginners' classes, and if there aren't any persuading someone to start one.

Once you're fit enough to get in shape, don't feel that you have to opt for jogging or cycling or swimming. There's no reason why you can't take up any active sport you enjoy – tennis, squash, badminton, basketball, even football – since obviously enjoyment is very important in motivating you to keep going and boredom is one of the main factors in the high drop-out rate in most keep-fit classes.

But perhaps one reason why jogging has become so popular, especially among people who've never been 'sporty', is that it's non-competitive. Many of the GETTING IN SHAPE participants said they would not have become involved in the project if it had been competitive – possibly a hangover from school days when not to be 'good at games' was to be an object of ridicule, not only from your peers but from the PE teacher too.

Another reason for the popularity of jogging is that it is so easy to take up. You don't have to pay a fortune to join a club, or, with the exception of decent running shoes, to acquire the necessary kit. You don't have to book a court days in advance, you don't have to rely on lots of other people, and you don't have to devote the best part of every Saturday or every Wednesday evening to it to get the full benefit. If you come home from work and feel like going for a run you can just put on your gear and go. And within thirty to forty minutes you can be home again, showered, changed, and ready to get on with the rest of the evening.

Almost all the GETTING IN SHAPE aerobes found that belonging to a group was extremely important in keeping them going, even though they ran three times a week on their own and only once with the group. With running the second most popular participation sport after angling, it could hardly be easier these days to join a fun-running group. There are literally thousands of them up and down the country, based in pubs, sports clubs, or even offices, and if by any chance there isn't one near you, then it's very easy to get one started. Initially, you don't need a headquarters or even a changing-room – people can arrive ready changed with something warm to put on afterwards, or can even change in their cars. Fellow joggers can be recruited by putting a notice up in the local pub, on the office noticeboard, or even in the local paper, inviting anyone interested to meet at a certain time in a certain place. Will Chapman, administrative director of GETTING IN SHAPE, who has vast experience of setting up funrunning groups, suggests that the meeting place is close to a convenient pub and the time is one that allows you to finish during opening hours! 'The social side is important and you need somewhere to go after you've finished training to talk about it, and basically forge the bonds that will actually keep people coming back week after week. I do know of one group that has made its base in a local teashop, and its members seem very happy with that. But I think most people prefer a pub!'

In Will Chapman's experience the most successful groups are those that have grown organically, with structure and organisation developing spontaneously as the members felt the need for it, rather than having it imposed on them right from the start. Some groups don't even have a name – they're just known as the lot that meets in the Queen's Head car park every Tuesday – until someone decides it would be more convenient to call themselves the Queen's Head Runners. If you're looking for a name for your group, choose something that isn't too intimidating like the Stragglers, the Trotters, or the Tail-Enders, rather than the Harriers which makes it sound like an élite running club.

Ideally, you will find other people in the group wanting to take an active role in the organisation – organising group entries in local fun runs, for example, or, as the numbers increase, starting a newsletter to keep everyone in touch with what's going on. All these activities help to establish the group's identity and are obviously done with greater enthusiasm by people who dream them up themselves than by those who've had the task thrust on them by the committee.

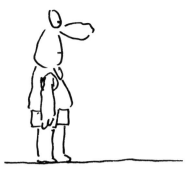 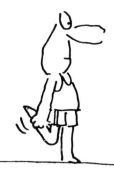

In fact, initiative should be greatly encouraged. During GETTING IN SHAPE, the participants were not able to express themselves in this way, since they were part of a complex scientific study, and while the trainers were told to allow any such developments to evolve naturally, they were instructed not to give any active encouragement.

Although one of the attractions of fun-running for many people is that it is largely non-competitive, it became very clear from GETTING IN SHAPE that most people do need a goal to aim at. The initial goal for most people in the project was to get in shape, but since many of them had reached their peak of fitness after the first six months or so, some other sort of motivation was needed. For the anaerobes that did present a real problem, for the only option open to them if they were going to keep within the design of the experiment was to increase the number of exercise circuits they did or increase the number of exercises within each circuit.

For the aerobes, though, it was much easier, and the groups were able to set tangible goals for themselves – the *Sunday Times* Fun Run, the Paris–Versailles 10-kilometre race, a half marathon somewhere and so on. There are now literally thousands of 'citizen races' around the country to choose from – everything from 2.5-mile fun runs, through to 10 kilometres, 10 miles, half marathons, marathons and even super marathons of 50 miles plus!

Choose a target race that is realistic for most of the people in your group, both in terms of length and the amount of time you have to train for it. The 'Fun Runner '82' project showed that it was perfectly possible to take unfit beginners and train them from scratch for the 2.5-mile *Sunday Times* Fun Run in five months.

Finding the right trainers is obviously the key to success in a project like this. You might be tempted to try and rope in experienced PE teachers or instructors, but that would be a mistake. People who have never been unfit themselves often find it hard to understand that for absolute beginners it is impossible to run for more than a minute or two initially, and they aren't just being feeble. As GETTING IN SHAPE showed very clearly, the ideal trainers were people who were comparative beginners themselves and remembered only too well what it was like to be totally out of condition!

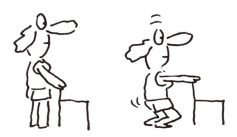

Ideally, for a group of ten beginners, Will Chapman believes you need two trainers: one of average ability and one 'plodder'. If the group is mixed, then preferably there should be one trainer of each sex. Some women find it easier to start in a single-sex group to get over the unease many of them feel about appearing red-faced and sweaty in front of men. But Will Chapman is convinced that the sooner they are absorbed into a mixed group, and preferably a family group, the better. 'Some of the most successful fun-running groups are those which have always encouraged families to join by organising sports days with events for everybody. If wives and children are taking part instead of standing at the roadside watching Dad go by twice an hour they're much more likely to be enthusiastic about it, and if they are then he's more likely to remain enthusiastic too.'

It became clear from GETTING IN SHAPE that a number of people found the fact that they were being monitored medically very reassuring. Obviously, it wouldn't be practical for small fun-running groups to set up something similar, but it's a good idea if possible to recruit a local GP if not as a runner, then as an interested by-stander. Ideally, it should be someone prepared to give beginners a check-up to make sure there aren't any serious medical problems, and who would be sympathetic to the odd sports injury. It doesn't do a great deal for your motivation to be told that the only cure for your sore Achilles' tendon is to give up running altogether!

Of course, many sports injuries can be avoided with proper preparation. Every session should start with at least ten or fifteen minutes of warm-up exercises with gentle stretching of Achilles' tendons, calves, hamstrings, abductors, and short bursts of jogging on the spot to get the heart working harder. The very first group session should involve a maximum of ten minutes jogging, and absolute beginners should be encouraged to walk whenever they get breathless, even if it means one of the trainers walking with them. Non-competitive or not, no one likes to be the first – or the only one – to give up, so the idea should be encouraged from the start that what matters is progressing at their own pace and that what other people are doing is irrelevant. It will soon become clear that some members of the group are progressing faster than others, and they should be assigned to trainers accordingly. It may well happen that people will pair off naturally with someone who runs at the same pace as they do, and if it doesn't, then the trainers should encourage it. Running the same route on your own week after week can become pretty boring, but if you've got someone you can chat with while you're running, you really don't notice the distance.

At the end of every session, group members should be encouraged to spend ten minutes or so 'warming down' and in particular, gently stretching their muscles – rather than simply pulling on a tracksuit and hurrying in for a pint. Leave them with instructions to repeat what they've just done every other day, and not to try and do more.

At the next session increase the amount of time you spend jogging and walking by a couple of minutes and no more. 'It

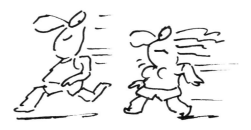

really does pay to build up the time spent jogging and the distances covered very gradually,' said Will Chapman, 'making sure that the pace is always easy. We always say that if you can't chat comfortably to the person with whom you're running, then you're going too fast. In a sense, it is self-limiting. If you set off too fast, you'll limit the distance you can run. If you want to up the distance from three miles to four, say, you'll obviously have to drop your pace.'

Once people become more confident, and are no longer afraid of looking silly, many of them may enjoy an element of competition. Certainly the sports days organised for the GETTING IN SHAPE participants were attended with great enthusiasm and thoroughly enjoyed, perhaps because people were competing in teams not as individuals. On a regular basis, and for small clubs especially, handicap races are probably the best idea because, if the handicaps are properly worked out, then even the slowest runner in the group who puts in a bit of extra effort can win.

THE PROGRAMME

GETTING IN SHAPE demonstrated very clearly that aerobic and anaerobic exercise offer different but equally valuable benefits, so the ideal programme for people who are out of shape but who want to do something about it is a combination of the two.

This programme, devised by Malcom Emery, formerly of the West London Institute and now of City Health Care, is based on the experience gleaned from GETTING IN SHAPE. It offers a choice of aerobic exercise – walking, cycling, exercise-cycling and swimming as well as jogging – and is designed to take no more than a couple of hours a week (or less if you decide to get your aerobic exercise by walking or cycling to work) so that even the busiest person can fit it in.

Use the two exercise programmes together, either doing the anaerobic exercises before your aerobic sessions, or doing the two programmes on alternate days. Both exercise programmes are graded 'Beginners', 'Intermediate' and 'Advanced', and you should not progress to the next level until you are ready to do so on both.

Always warm up properly at the start of every exercise session. Start with two or three minutes' gentle jogging on the spot to get your heart and lungs working harder. Then do the following exercises.

ARM CIRCLING
Stand with your arms at your sides and your legs slightly apart. Move both arms backwards together, making full, slow circles. Try to cover the full range of movement, and to feel slight stretching sensations in the backs of your shoulders as you

extend to the extremities of your reach. Do not make any quick, jerky movements. Do 5 full circles backwards, 5 forwards and then repeat.

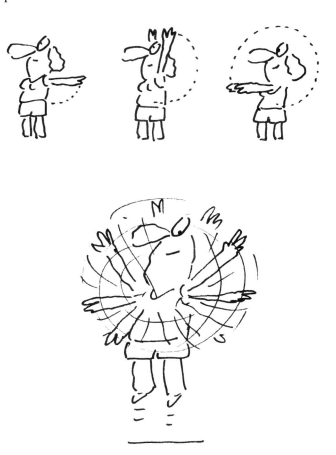

BEND AND STRETCH
Stand with your feet shoulder-width apart, keeping your knees slightly bent. Bend your body until your hands are near or on the floor between your legs. Slowly straighten your whole body,

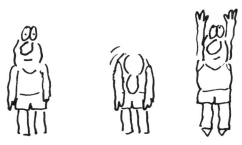

pushing your hips forward and keeping your shoulders back. Arch your neck and back, raising your arms all the way over your head and bend your head back. Attempt to cover the full range of movement and to feel slight stretching sensations in your back, stomach, shoulders and backs of legs. As you return to the starting position, keep your knees bent. Avoid making any quick, jerky movements. Repeat the exercise 10 times.

KNEE TUCKS

Sit on the floor with your legs straight and together in front of you. Place your hands on your thighs. Bend your right knee up, clasp both arms around it and gently draw your leg into your chest until you can feel the tightness in your knee. Release and lower. Repeat with the left leg. Do 10 repetitions with each leg.

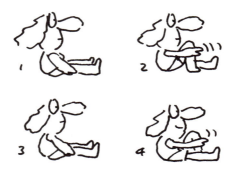

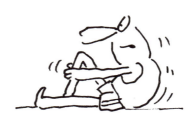

HALF SQUATS

Stand behind a chair (or other suitable support) with your feet shoulder-width apart. Stand upright and support both your hands on the chair back. Keeping your back straight and holding onto the chair back, slowly bend your knees and lower your body to a half-squat position. Hold this for 2 seconds and then return to the upright position. Shake your legs. Repeat this exercise 10 times.

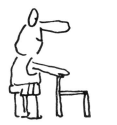 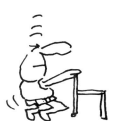

Rest for 60 seconds and prepare to commence your appropriate training programme.

It's also important that you 'warm down' for a few minutes at the end of every exercise session, with a little gentle jogging on the spot and some stretching exercises. However tempting it may be to dive straight into a shower as soon as you've finished, allow your body time to cool down a little first. Don't exercise immediately after a heavy meal or if you have a bad cold, 'flu or a temperature. A mild cold or sore throat, once the initial symptoms have passed, shouldn't stop you exercising, nor should minor ailments like backache or bowel trouble. If you start to feel worse while you're exercising, then stop.

Take it gently – it's very easy to get carried away with enthusiasm when you start and do more than the programme prescribes. That way you are liable to damage muscles or joints unused to such exertion. In extreme cases you could put an intolerable strain on your heart, or, which is more likely, you'll just feel so terrible that the new tracksuit and training shoes, along with all your good intentions, will get thrown into a cupboard and forgotten.

ANAEROBIC EXERCISE

THE EXERCISES

WALL PUSH-AWAYS

Stand at arms' length from the wall, feet together, hands flat on the wall and arms straight. Keeping your whole body in a straight line, lean forwards, bending your arms, until your nose touches the wall. Push yourself upright again by straightening your arms.

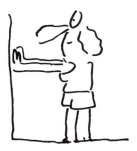 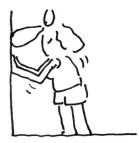 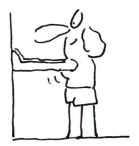

SEMI PRESS-UPS

Go down on your hands and knees, with your arms at right angles to the floor and your thighs at forty-five degrees. Keeping your back straight, bend your arms until your chin touches the floor, then straighten your arms again.

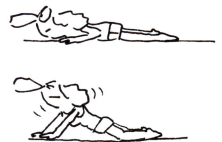

LEG RAISES

Lie flat, with the small of your back pushed well into the floor and your pelvis tilted slightly upwards to avoid straining your back. With your knees slightly bent, lift your legs about 18″ off the ground, either one at a time or together according to the level you are on. You should feel the pull in your abdomen, *not* in your back.

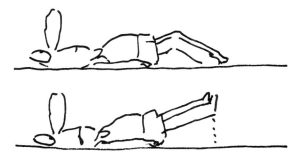

PRESS-UPS

Lie face downwards, placing your hands flat on the floor underneath your shoulders. Push upwards until your arms are quite straight, keeping only your toes in contact with the floor. Maintaining your body in a straight, rigid position, lower yourself gently until your chin, chest and hips touch the ground at the same time.

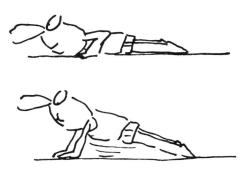

STAR JUMPS
Stand upright with your feet together. Bend your knees slightly, jump into the star position, then into your starting position.

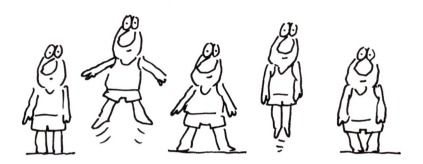

STEP-UPS
Stand in front of a bench or step 12–15" high. Step onto the bench to achieve an upright, straight-legged position. Then step down, back to your starting position.

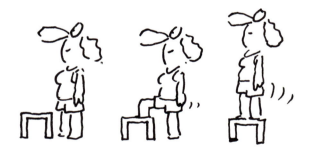

SQUAT THRUSTS
Squat on the ground, your hands resting on the ground just in front of your feet. Jump both legs back until they are stretched out straight behind you. Then jump them in to just behind your hands to resume your starting position.

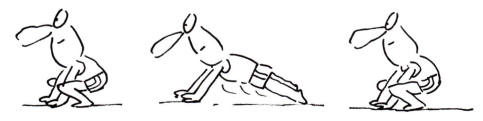

SIT-UPS

Lie as for leg raises, with your hands crossed on your chest. Keeping your feet on the floor, sit up. Again, you should feel the pull in your abdomen, *not* in your back.

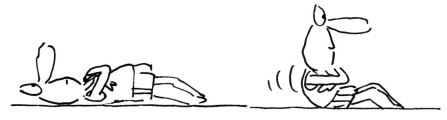

BACK RAISES

Lie on your front, with your hands clasped at the back of your neck. Raise the top half of your body as far off the floor as you can comfortably manage, then lower it again.

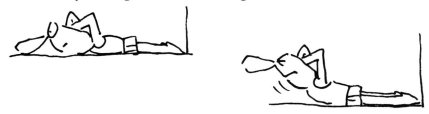

SHOPPING-BAG CURL LIFTS

Put 5 lb (a bag of potatoes for instance) in a plastic carrier bag and hold it with your palm facing forwards and your arm straight down by your side. Keeping your arm close to your side, bring your hand up to your shoulder and then lower it at the same speed. (In other words, make the muscles work: don't just let the bag drop!)

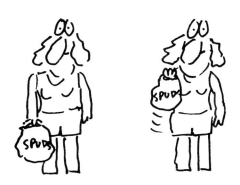

SHOPPING-BAG OUTWARD LIFTS

Hold the shopping bag with your arm straight down by your side, but this time with the back of your hand facing forward. Keeping it straight, raise your arm to shoulder level, and then lower it again at the same speed.

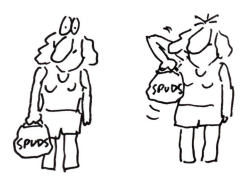

BEGINNERS: LEVEL 1

10 Wall push-aways
10 Leg raises with each leg
10 Shopping-bag curl lifts
10 Squat thrusts (only move your feet forward about 12". Don't try to bring your knees up to your chest)
10 Back raises
10 Shopping-bag outward lifts

When you can complete two circuits comfortably, move on to –

BEGINNERS: LEVEL 2

The same exercises as Level 1 except –
10 Semi press-ups instead of wall push-aways
10 Leg raises, 5 with each leg and 5 with both legs

Add one repetition to each exercise until you are doing 15 of each. When you can complete 3 circuits comfortably, move on to –

INTERMEDIATE: LEVEL 1

15 Full press-ups
15 Star jumps
15 Leg raises with both legs together
15 Shopping-bag curl lifts
15 Full squat thrusts
15 Back raises
15 Shopping-bag outward lifts
15 Step-ups (15 with the right leg leading, 15 with the left)

Do the exercises briskly, with a ninety-second rest between each set. When you can do each exercise set in thirty seconds, move on to –

INTERMEDIATE: LEVEL 2

The same exercises as Level 1 except –
15 Sit-ups instead of 15 Leg raises

Do as many repetitions of each exercise as you can in twenty seconds with a ninety-second rest between each set. When you can do 15 repetitions in twenty seconds, move on to –

ADVANCED: LEVEL 1

Do as many repetitions as you can in thirty seconds, with a ninety-second rest between each set. When you can do 20 repetitions in thirty seconds, move on to –

ADVANCED: LEVEL 2

Do as many repetitions as you can in thirty seconds, with a sixty-second rest between each set.

AEROBIC EXERCISE

Choose the kind of exercise you find most appealing and easiest to fit into your daily routine. The programmes are interchangeable, but if you do switch, then you should drop down five levels to give the different muscle groups a chance to develop. The exception is swimming, which demands much more skill than running, cycling or walking, so you should start at the beginning.

AEROBIC TRAINING SCHEDULE

DAY:	1	2	3	4	5	6	7	TOTAL
LEVEL 1	5 min	Rest	5 min	Rest	Rest	7 min	Rest	17 min
LEVEL 2	7 min	Rest	7 min	Rest	Rest	10 min	Rest	24 min
LEVEL 3	10 min	Rest	10 min	Rest	Rest	12 min	Rest	32 min
LEVEL 4	12 min	Rest	12 min	Rest	Rest	15 min	Rest	39 min
LEVEL 5	15 min	Rest	15 min	Rest	Rest	18 min	Rest	48 min
LEVEL 6	15 min	Rest	18 min	Rest	Rest	20 min	Rest	53 min
LEVEL 7	18 min	Rest	20 min	Rest	Rest	22 min	Rest	60 min
LEVEL 8	18 min	Rest	20 min	Rest	10 min	22 min	Rest	70 min
LEVEL 9	20 min	Rest	22 min	Rest	10 min	25 min	Rest	77 min
LEVEL 10	20 min	Rest	25 min	Rest	10 min	28 min	Rest	83 min
LEVEL 11	20 min	Rest	27 min	Rest	12 min	32 min	Rest	91 min
LEVEL 12	20 min	Rest	30 min	Rest	12 min	35 min	Rest	97 min
LEVEL 13	20 min	Rest	30 min	Rest	15 min	38 min	Rest	103 min
LEVEL 14	20 min	Rest	30 min	Rest	15 min	40 min	Rest	105 min

If you are doing your aerobic and anaerobic exercise on different days, you should not only do the warm-up routine before you go out for a run or a bicycle ride, but the following stretching exercises as well. They are all 'passive' stretches, the safest kind because they are self-limiting – you can only stretch the muscles as far as they will go naturally and no further. For that reason, you should hold the stretch still for ten seconds. You should *not* bounce.

EXERCISE A   For the Calves and Achilles' Tendons

Stand facing the wall, hands flat on it, arms straight. Put your left foot about 18" behind the right. Keeping your left heel flat on the floor and your left leg straight, bend your right knee until you feel the stretch in your left calf. Hold it for ten seconds then repeat with the other leg.

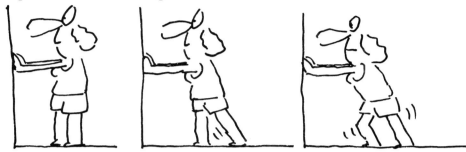

Muscles must *always* be stretched individually.

EXERCISE B   For the Soleus (the deeper calf muscle)

Start in the same position as for exercise A, only this time, bend your front leg, keeping the heel flat on the floor, and your weight forward. The back leg is only there for support, so it doesn't matter if it bends or the heel comes off the floor. You should feel the stretch deep in your calf. Hold it for ten seconds and repeat with the other leg.

EXERCISE C   For the Shins (the anterior tibials)

Kneel with your knees about 6" apart, and the tops of your feet as flat on the floor as possible. Sit back on your heels until you feel a stretch in your shins. Don't try and hold a position halfway down as it puts too much of a strain on your thigh muscles. Hold the stretch for ten seconds. Straighten up and repeat it.

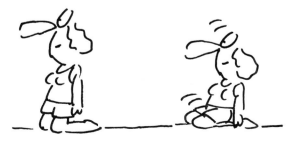

EXERCISE D   For Thigh Muscles (quadriceps)

Stand straight, bend your right leg and take hold of your right foot or ankle with your right hand. Keeping your body straight, gently pull your foot backwards until you feel the stretch in your thigh. Ideally, your right thigh should be parallel to your left. Hold it for ten seconds and repeat with the other leg.

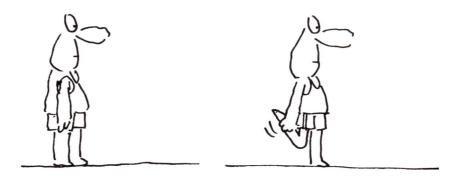

EXERCISE E   For Hamstrings

Stand upright and put your right leg onto a low stool, rail or stair. Keep it straight and lean forward slightly until you feel the stretch at the back of your thigh. Hold it for ten seconds and repeat with the other leg.

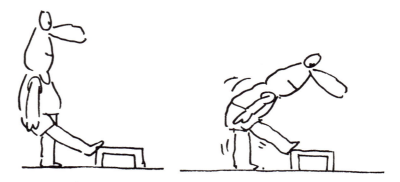

EXERCISE F	For the Abductors (the muscles inside your thighs)

Stand with your feet about 18" apart, then swing your hips to the left and when you feel the stretch in the inside of your right thigh hold it for ten seconds. Then swing your hips out to the right until you feel the stretch in the left thigh and hold it for ten seconds.

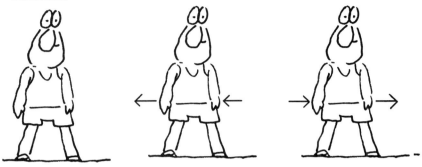

EXERCISE G	For the Glutei (muscles in the buttocks)

Stand upright, bend your right knee and pull it into your chest with both hands. When you feel the stretch in your buttocks, hold it for ten seconds. Repeat with the left leg.

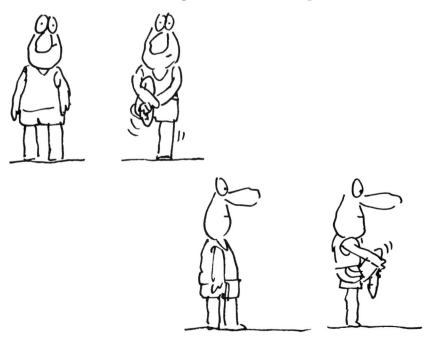

EXERCISE H	For the Hip Abductors and the Iliotibial Tract (band of fibrous tissue linking upper part of thigh with outside of knee)

Sit on the floor, bend your right knee and place your right foot on the floor outside your left knee. Turn your upper body to the right and bending your left arm, push your left elbow gently against the outside of your right knee. (It's much less complicated than it sounds!) Hold it for ten seconds. Repeat with the left leg bent.

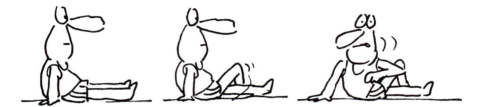

5

SPORTS INJURIES

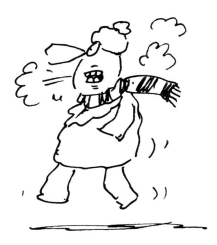

Among some members of the medical profession, jogging, fun-running and even aerobic dancing have acquired a bad name simply because of the number of injuries they cause which require treatment in GPs' surgeries, hospital casualty and physiotherapy departments. But, according to David Lindsay, a physiotherapist with wide experience of sports injuries and himself a keen runner, most injuries are avoidable if you follow a few basic guidelines.

Don't try to do too much too soon. Your body needs time to adjust to increased activity, so build up gradually. It's a good idea to join a group because other members will be able to advise you on a sensible training schedule and help you stick to it. Even when you are training regularly, increase the distances you run very gradually (no more than 10% in a week) and don't make any sudden changes in your running pattern. If you're used to running on flat ground, don't suddenly start running up 1-in-3 hills!

Warm up and warm down. Cold, tight muscles are much more prone to injury than warm, stretched muscles. Before you start exercising, you should *always* warm up with a few simple exercises and stretches (see page 76 for simple exercises, 87 for stretches). Just as important, though it's something that is often neglected, you should always warm *down* too, and stretching your muscles again at the end of a session will help prevent stiffness and soreness the following day. Each session should last about fifteen minutes – longer if it's a particularly cold day or you are starting to get in shape again after a long lay-off.

Wear suitable clothing. The right clothing is important too. In winter you need several layers of light clothes to trap your body heat and keep your muscles warm, rather than one thick layer which will impede your movements. In very cold weather you may need a hat, and you'll certainly need gloves. Even jogging slowly can increase the 'wind-chill factor' and joggers have been known to suffer from frost-bitten fingers. In summer you'll need cotton shorts and a vest, preferably a mesh vest which allows the air to circulate and perspiration to evaporate which in turn has a cooling effect on the body. Man-made fibres which don't 'breathe' make you sweat more, and dehydrating – losing too much fluid – can be dangerous. In very hot weather you need a hat to keep the sun off the back of your neck and protection for your shoulders to avoid sunstroke and sunburn.

Decent footwear is vital. By far and away the most important factor in avoiding injury, David Lindsay believes, is choosing the right running shoes. '75% of all running injuries result to some extent from wearing the wrong shoes – and that is a conservative estimate! Badly fitting shoes can not only injure your feet. They can also cause problems with your shins, Achilles' tendons, knees, hamstrings, hips and even your back!' His advice is not to go to a department store or chain of general shoe shops, or even general sports stores but to a specialist running shop. There the staff are likely to be runners themselves and will be keen to help you find the right shoes. Again, if you join a group, the other members will be able to recommend the best local shop, and even if it means making a special journey to a nearby town it is well worth it. A good shop will let you try running outside on the pavement, wearing the shoes. Obviously, trying them on sitting down or just walking around inside the shop won't tell you whether they're going to be comfortable when you run.

The well-known brand-names like Nike, New Balance, Etonic, Reebok are all reliable, but they all produce so many different shoes that the name alone is no guarantee that they will be right for you. Nor is the price. Although a good pair of shoes will cost you at least £30, that doesn't mean that a pair costing

£60 will be twice as good. The main points to watch out for when you're buying shoes are:

a) They should have plenty of cushioning under the heel – that is where most of the force goes when you land. If you push your thumb hard into the rubber, there should be a good, springy recoil when you let go. Heels that are too high can cause injury – they throw you off-balance and you can 'fall off' your shoes. The sole should be flexible.

b) The shoes should grip you firmly but comfortably round the heel so that your foot doesn't move from side to side as you run. There has been a lot of controversy about heel tabs and the damage they can do to the Achilles' tendon. If they are rigid and hard, as they are on many cheap, chain-store training shoes, they can cause injury, but on reputable makes the tabs are soft and well padded and shouldn't cause problems.

c) There should be ample support for the arch of your foot. If your arches do not rest on the arch supports you'll find they soon begin to ache as you run. More important, the lack of support could lead to a number of injuries. If the shoes are all right in every other respect you can usually solve this problem by fitting arch supports.

Socks should be of thin cotton (chain stores like Marks and Spencer and even Sainsbury's sell perfectly good ones at under half the price of brand-named running socks!) and should fit properly – not tight, but not so loose that the fabric forms folds on top of your toes.

Obviously, when you start exercising, muscles that have been doing only the bare minimum for years are bound to feel stiff and even sore the next day. 'Warming down' should help, as will hot baths, but if you really are very stiff then try a gentle form of exercise for a few days – swimming or cycling – until the stiffness goes and then start training again gradually.

Even if you are a beginner, you should be able to distinguish between stiffness or soreness and pain – and pain is something you should *never* ignore. Whether it is sharp and sudden, or a dull, persistent ache, pain is nature's way of telling you to stop! When a seasoned runner talks about going through the pain barrier, he or she means the psychological barrier he reaches when his body is telling him it's tired and has had enough. He does *not* mean that he would carry on running in spite of pain in a hamstring or Achilles' tendon. If you carry on running with a minor injury, it's more likely to become a major injury than it is to go away.

Same with cramp in a muscle. It is usually the result of a muscle tightening because it has been worked into a fatigued state. If you go on working it, it will tighten still further and possibly tear. So stop what you're doing and gently stretch it. To help prevent cramp make sure that you drink plenty of liquid, but don't start taking salt tablets unless your doctor advises you to do so, and do stretching exercises regularly before and after you train.

If you do injure yourself in spite of taking sensible precautions then you need medical advice, preferably from a GP or physio-therapist experienced in sports injuries and sympathetic to runners. Simply being told to give up running altogether isn't helpful! It may well be that the injury is only minor and there is no treatment for it other than rest, but it's important that a doctor sees it to be sure that it isn't something more serious. With almost every injury, serious or not, a simple First-Aid routine can help – Ice and Elevation.

Ice pressed against the injured part stimulates the flow of blood and therefore of healing white corpuscles through the muscle, reduces internal bleeding, and helps reduce swelling. You can either wrap the injured part in a towel dipped in iced water, or press ice cubes in a plastic bag or a small packet of frozen vegetables against it. Don't put ice directly onto your skin as it can 'burn'. Cover it with a towel or tea towel first, and hold the ice in place for ten to fifteen minutes.

Rest the injured leg as much as possible by raising your foot above your hip – lying on the sofa, for instance, with your lower leg supported by soft cushions. Although the cardiovascular system is designed to pump blood uphill, against gravity, that isn't true of fluid produced by an injured joint or muscle. Keeping your leg up will help prevent the fluid from gathering and causing swelling.

Obviously, you will have to give up running, though for how long will depend on what you have injured and how badly. That doesn't mean you can't do any exercise. With some injuries, you can cycle, and with almost all, you can swim, because the injured muscle or joint isn't taking your weight.

INJURIES

TOES

Blisters are caused by shoes that don't fit properly or socks that are too large so that folds of the fabric rub your toes.
Remedy. In the short term, treat them with surgical spirit. In the long term, get proper fitting shoes and socks.

Black toe nails. Black bruising under the nail of the big toes can be caused by shoes that are too tight, or where the toe nail is repeatedly catching on the stitching of the shoe and being pulled back, causing bleeding under the nail.
Remedy. Change your shoes.

Stress fractures of the big toe are caused by over-use.
Remedy. Rest for between six weeks and two months.

Metatarsalgia, an acute pain in the forefoot resulting from inflamed nerves in the ball of the foot; is usually caused by a structural problem, such as very high arches.
Remedy. Rest and make sure your shoes have adequate arch supports. Fit additional felt pads if necessary.

ARCHES

Painful or sore arches are usually caused by inadequate arch supports in your shoes.
Remedy. Fit arch supports to your shoes. To help strengthen your arches try gripping a pencil under your toes and holding it for five seconds. Relax and repeat the exercise up to 20 times a day.

HEELS

Blisters are caused by ill-fitting shoes that allow your heel to move around as you run, or are too tight, or by heel tabs that are too hard.
Remedy. Change your shoes, or cut off the heel tabs if that is the problem. Treat blisters with surgical spirit. Don't prick them in case they become infected and take longer to heal.

ANKLES

Torn ligaments are caused by twisting your ankle on an uneven surface or tripping in a pot hole. Although most other injuries come on gradually, this one is instant.

Remedy. Although First Aid – Ice and Elevation – will help ease the pain and possibly limit the damage, you will need professional treatment – strapping up, rest, and then physiotherapy to re-educate the muscles around the ankle to protect it.

ACHILLES' TENDONS

The Achilles' tendon, which attaches the muscles of the lower leg to the heel, becomes inflamed, painful and tender to the touch just above the heel usually as a result of over-use – either increasing the distances you are running too quickly, or starting to do hill runs without enough preparation. Pain higher up is usually the result of heel tabs or high backs of your shoes digging into the tendon.

Remedy. In the short term, treat it with ice and rest it. Achilles' tendon injuries are slow to heal, so it really isn't worth taking chances. In the long term try putting heel-raises in your shoes. By lifting the heel a little you are putting less strain on the Achilles' tendon. If the problem is caused by heel tabs, either cut them off, or cut down each side of the tab about an inch so it no longer digs into the tendon. Do Stretching Exercise A regularly before and after training.

CALVES

Calf muscles, which produce the spring necessary for running and jumping, seem to be among the first to degenerate when you are unfit, and so are particularly vulnerable to injury once you start getting in shape. Women who always wear high-heeled shoes are even more prone to injury because those muscles don't get stretched in everyday life and so tend to be short and tight. Simply putting on a pair of flat running shoes, never mind actually running, puts the muscles under much more tension than they are used to. (Before you start running, wear your running shoes around the house for a few hours at a time to get the muscles used to the new alignment.) Injury to the calf muscles is usually caused by strenuous exercise when they are cold, tight or fatigued. The site of the injury will be painful to touch and you will find walking painful.

Remedy. In the short term, apply ice, and as soon as the pain allows start gentle stretching exercises. In this case, movement actually helps the healing process.

As a preventative measure, do Stretching Exercises A and B every day as well as just before and after every training session.

SHINS

Shin splints, the painful swelling of the muscles of the shin, common in novice runners, usually results from over-use, from running on your toes or the balls of your feet, weak arches or inadequate support for the arches in your shoes. The muscles for the feet and ankles start in the shins, so if the arch isn't properly supported the foot rolls inwards as it lands ('over-pronating' is the technical term), putting additional strain on the muscles and ligaments of the shin by pulling them diagonally.

Remedy. In the short term, Ice and Elevation and rest for anything between two and six weeks. In the long term, correct your running style if necessary, making sure you land heel first. Check that your shoes are providing adequate support for your arches, and when you start training again run only on level ground and build up distances very gradually. You should also do Stretching Exercise C regularly before and after training.

KNEES

Ligament injuries, which can be painful either inside or outside the knee, are often caused by a faulty running style which makes the foot either over-pronate (roll inwards on landing) or over-supinate (roll outwards), both of which can put strain on a ligament.

Remedy. In the short term, Ice and Elevation. In the long term, if you are inclined to pronate, make sure that your shoes give your arches enough support.

Runner's Knee (Retro-patellar arthrosis) is a vague, dull ache on the kneecap which gets worse when you walk upstairs, run or walk up a slope or get up after sitting down for some time. It's caused by over-use, or by problems with the alignment of the lower leg.

Remedy. In the short term, Ice and Elevation. In the long term, make sure your shoes fit properly, since the position of your feet dictates the alignment of the lower leg; and strengthen the muscles by straightening your leg while you're sitting on a chair, locking the knee and holding it for ten seconds. Relax and repeat 10 times.

Iliotibial tract friction causes a sharp, stinging pain on the outside of your knee where the iliotibial tract, which runs down the outside of your thigh between your hip and your shin, is attached to the bone. It is usually caused by over-use, hill-running without adequate preparation, running on a heavily cambered road which puts strain on the 'down' leg, or choosing a long, circular route which means you are always turning in the same direction and putting more stress on one knee and hip alignment.

Remedy. In the short term, Ice and Elevation. In the long term, to prevent it recurring, choose a non-circular route, and do Stretching Exercise H regularly before and after training. With some knee injuries, swimming may not be a good idea. The leg action in breast stroke could aggravate the injury, so try it and see. If the pain feels worse, stop.

HAMSTRINGS

A strain or even tear of the hamstrings, the group of muscles at the back of your thigh, is usually caused by over-use, especially when the muscle is cold or tight (if you haven't warmed up properly at the start of exercise) or fatigued (if you've actually gone on too long). It can also be caused by a change in your usual running pattern – running on an uneven surface or on a cambered road. Even wearing different shoes can cause it.

Remedy. In the short term, ice, compression and rest. You must make sure the injury is fully healed and the muscle fully flexible again before you start running, otherwise you are likely to damage it again. In the long term, make sure you do Stretching Exercise E regularly before and after training.

HIPS

A deep, dull ache in the deep-seated hip flexor muscles at the front of the hip (those that put the thigh forward) or in the tensor fascia lata, which goes over the hip bone and is connected to the iliotibial tract, is usually caused by over-use – running much longer distances than you are used to, increasing your speed, hill-running, or possibly by running a circular route. A similar pain in the piriformis (the point of the hip) can be caused by over-pronation – the foot rolling inwards as it lands.

Remedy. In the short term, ice and rest. In the long term, make sure your shoes have adequate arch supports, and do Stretching Exercise H regularly before and after training.

BACK

Back problems, which can be felt as pain in the hips or buttocks, are often caused by running on hard surfaces with insufficient cushioning in your shoes, which jars your spine. This is potentially quite dangerous because it can cause compression of the nerves and loss of sensation in your legs. If you have any persistent dull pain in your lower back, buttocks, hips, upper legs, with or without shooting pains, or any numbness, you should see a doctor right away.

Remedy. Make sure your shoes have sufficient cushioning, and when you start running again stick to flat, soft surfaces until your body adjusts.

6

SOME FINAL WORDS

There is no doubt that the GETTING IN SHAPE project changed many of its participants' lives in a quite profound and unexpected way. Many of them showed an improvement physiologically, but for most of them that was less important than the psychological changes they experienced.

'My general sense of well-being and self-confidence has increased, but most of all my outlook on life has changed. I feel twenty years younger!'

'I think of GETTING IN SHAPE as the Year of Great Joy. It's changed my life, and it's the best £100 investment I ever made!'

'I have almost become hooked on the idea that physical fitness alters your attitudes to almost everything – food, play, work, sex, tolerance of others – all to the benefit of oneself and one's friends.'

These sentiments, expressed by three participants, were shared by the vast majority of those who took part.

Once the project came to an end most of the groups disbanded. A few did carry on for a while at the behest of members who felt that they needed the group in order to keep going, and one group, in north London, is still going strong, having drawn in partners, friends and colleagues of the original participants too.

Naturally, some people have stopped exercising regularly, but, as one man put it, they know that any time they decide they want to get in shape again they can do it. For many other people exercise is now so much a part of their daily routine that they can't imagine life without it. Some have taken up a sport they used to play in their youth, others have started something new. And some are still running, going out on their own two or three evenings a week, or taking part in fun runs and 'citizen races' in this country and abroad. Indeed, there have been GETTING IN SHAPERS in every London Marathon since the project began.

At a time when it has become fashionable in some quarters to knock exercise as boring, obsessive, masochistic and hazardous to health, it is reassuring to learn from the GETTING IN SHAPE project that not only is exercise very good for you physically, mentally and emotionally, but that practically everybody who chooses to do it can get fit.

APPENDIX 1

FOR THE SCIENTIFICALLY MINDED

This study involved thousands of measurements that can be compared and contrasted in many ways. They have been summarised in a report (obtainable from Brompton Hospital) which essentially said the following things:

a) A group of 174 subjects were recruited from Londoners, aged thirty to fifty-eight, who read the *Sunday Times*, felt they were under-exercised and were prepared to pay £100 to take part in a year-long progressive physical training programme and to be subjected to exercise and lung-function tests at regular intervals.

b) Two of the 174 had to be rejected because of heart disease; the others included several people with minor cardiorespiratory disorders in the past but no recent history of significant heart or lung disease.

c) Preliminary studies on a group of fifty-one healthy people suggested the normal standards for lung function used by us at that time tended to underestimate the greatest volume of air they could blow out in one second (FEV1), the greatest volume they could blow out altogether (FVC), and the maximum volume of the lungs themselves (TLC). They also tended to underestimate the volume of use of blood in the lung (TLCO).

d) Another supporting study of, on average, 100 measurements of each lung-function variable in each of ten subjects over a period of two years showed the lung-volume variables were reproducible within ±3% and the lung-blood-volume variables reproducible within ±5%.

e) It also showed that the volume of lung that was effectively 'out of service' in the ten-second single-breath manoeuvre was 10.6 ± 2.8% of the total lung capacity in the same ten subjects studied on some 120 occasions on each subject over two years.

f) The subjects of the main GETTING IN SHAPE trial had the mean values and variability in each routine lung-function characteristic that were anticipated by the preliminary study. These suggest FEV1 and FVC predictions should be raised by some 10%, total lung-capacity predictions by 5%, and that useful blood volume of the lung (TLCO) predictions should be reduced by 7% in future studies on at least this type of Londoner. The predicted shortfall of VA on TLC (i.e. the volume of lung 'out of service') should be raised in this age group to $13.6 \pm 2\%$.

g) The group was divided into aerobic and anaerobic sets which were well matched for age, height, weight, sex and most routine measures of lung function, but differed very slightly in the aerobic capacities, total lung capacity and whole-lung carbon monoxide transfer, probably because of exercise preferences.

h) Both groups achieved close-to-predicted work loads and showed similar and standard variability in maximum loads between one subject and the next.

i) The statistical normality of their exercise and routine lung-function results allowed us to define new 'limits of normality' for this age group.

j) On exposure to a graded aerobic training programme for one year, the aerobic group showed a 7–14% increase in aerobic capacity, a 10–20 beats/minute reduction in heart rate at any given load and an unchanged ventilatory response to exertion.

k) The anaerobic group showed much slighter objective changes in the response to exercise.

l) Both groups showed small but definite improvements in lung function with training, most notably an increase in accessible gas volume (VA). The anaerobic group also showed an improvement in whole-lung carbon monoxide transfer (TLCO), probably reflecting an increase in pulmonary capillary blood volume. The improvements in lung function appeared to be related to need.

m) The improvements in aerobic capacity also appeared to be related to need.

At the end of the study, all of the participants were sent a questionnaire, regardless of whether they had completed the full twelve-month training programme or had dropped out earlier. This questionnaire was in six parts that concerned pre-project condition, motives for joining the scheme, the impact of training schedules, criticisms of the running of the project, physical effects of the programme and overall reactions to having participated. 104 replies were received. The results will be presented largely in a tabular form, where the figures speak for themselves. For questions where the answers are descriptive, the responses have been assessed qualitatively and added to a short summary of the tables. The comments are simply listed in order of frequency. Throughout the report the responses have been analysed in groups (by training and/or sex) only where it was thought to be relevant.

The questionnaire began by asking for some details of the participant's physical fitness before the project began (Table 1a). Their responses were summarised in Table 1b. Almost all (96%) had done some exercise since leaving school, most commonly swimming, squash and tennis, but including almost every sporting activity. However, 82% had not enjoyed or suffered any form of regular exercise of moderate intensity for at least five years (Fig. 1). At the time of beginning the study most subjects described themselves spontaneously in the following terms (in order of decreasing frequency): overweight; unfit; lethargic; sluggish; tired; okay; tired and depressed.

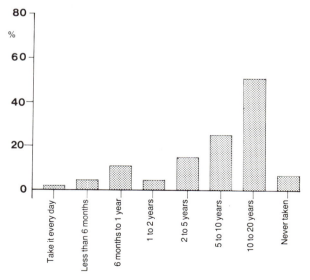

DELAY SINCE TAKING REGULAR EXERCISE

Figure 1   A histogram of the delay since taking regular exercise in the whole group.

22% sensed they were very unfit; 45% thought themselves to be 'slightly unfit'; 25% felt they were of average fitness; 7% believed themselves to be moderately fit; and 1% 'very fit'. This story of leaving school healthy, taking some part in sport thereafter and slowly sliding into 'unfitness', must be familiar to very many people in the thirty-to-sixty-year age range. It is interesting that at least 25% thought they were 'of average fitness'.

The intentions of the next questions were to discover some early influences on the subjects' attitudes towards exercise arising from physical education at school. 96% of the respondents had done PE at school. Of these, 75% said they had enjoyed it, 71% for either serious or friendly competition. The rest said it was for pleasure rather than competition. From these answers and the lists of activities which they favoured doing, there was evidently a tendency in the schools to present PE as a predominantly competitive activity. Although only one in four of the respondents felt that their experience of exercise at school had a lasting negative effect on them, three-quarters of the group had not done any regular physical activity since then. Those who felt that PE at school had affected them badly recall that they disliked competition, were bad at games and that the unsympathetic attitude of the staff further discouraged them from participating and made them feel inadequate and miserable. As a direct consequence of this they felt they had been put off any form of physical activity ever since due to the unpleasant associations and feelings of inferiority generated at school.

The next section of the questionnaire (Table 2a) concerned the motivation to join a project such as GETTING IN SHAPE, and the respondents' attitudes towards physical fitness at the time. The answers to the early part of this section (Table 2b) indicate that most of the participants were aware of the growing public interest in physical fitness in Britain and abroad, but that interest had not been sufficient to prompt them into any positive action until the *Sunday Times* advertisement introduced an opportunity to join a professionally supervised group. Those who had been persuaded to do something prior to the advertisement felt the influence came from this country rather than abroad. Those who had another sporting connection which encouraged them to join GETTING IN SHAPE mentioned the following:

a) 'My husband runs . . .'
b) 'Friends who ran . . .'
c) 'Skiing getting harder by the year . . .'
d) 'Cycling clubs . . .'
e) 'G. Cannon's *Dieting Makes You Fat* . . .'
f) 'Seeing Madge Sharples finish the London Marathon with-

out being out of breath . . .'
g) 'Watching people on TV . . .'

Many respondents felt that exercise reduced the risk of heart disease, and improved 'general health'. Evidently, the idea of using a supervised exercise programme was attractive to a large number of them. Most of the respondents (88% aerobic, 67% anaerobic) thought that both types of training would improve general fitness, though there was less certainty about anaerobic training. (33% anaerobic were 'unsure', Table 2b.)

The next section of the questionnaire (Table 3a) concerned subjects' expectations at the start of the scheme. Their replies are summarised in Table 3b. The first demand examined their reasons for choosing one type of training or the other. In the aerobic group, the motives for selecting this type of training were equally divided between a preference for aerobic exercise and a dislike for anaerobic exercise. In order of descending frequency the participants:
a) thought aerobic exercise easier.
b) had a great belief in jogging.
c) thought they could lose weight.
d) wanted to swim.
e) enjoyed running.
f) felt their characters more suited to endurance exercise.
g) thought aerobic exercise more beneficial to health.
h) disliked anaerobic training.
i) nearest training centre was aerobic.
j) felt they had more chance of acceptance to the scheme.

The anaerobic group seemed to choose their form of training by default rather than positive desire. Subjects:
a) did not want to run.
b) wanted to increase strength.
c) thought anaerobic exercise was less time-consuming.
d) thought aerobic exercise was harmful.
e) felt they had the wrong temperament for endurance exercise.
f) thought anaerobic exercise more interesting.
g) said anaerobic exercise was an 'unknown factor'.
h) felt they had more chance of acceptance to the scheme for anaerobic rather than aerobic exercise.
i) nearest training centre was anaerobic.
j) did not know the difference.

Two out of three respondents expected to lose weight during the project. More of these were aerobic than anaerobic. (Did images of thin runners and stout weight lifters influence them?)

Interestingly, more anaerobics expected to enjoy their chosen method of exercise than aerobics, despite the anaerobic subjects' apparent lack of confidence in the training method, indicated by answers to other questions.

Once the scheme had started, most people seemed to enjoy the group training sessions which, on the whole, made training much easier to complete. Their attitudes to the training pro-grammes were tested by the questions listed in Table 4a and their responses summarised in Table 4b. The aerobic group found their first few training sessions harder than did their anaerobic counterparts. More than half of both groups found the first training session enjoyable. Both groups also found that it was easier to train in company than alone. However, most of the participants exercised alone during the rest of the week and more than half of the women who ran felt anxious about doing so alone after dusk, although three quarters did so anyway.

Four out of five respondents said they never seriously con-sidered withdrawing from the project. The thing that was cited most often as being the driving force keeping them going to the end was a sense of commitment and determination to finish what they had started. There was also a strong loyalty to the group (i.e., training group), and to the trainers. The other main driving force was the improvement in their capacity to exercise and the fact that they were feeling better and were afraid of getting unfit again.

The influences driving the aerobic people were (in order of descending frequency):
a) Commitment.
b) Determination.
c) Enjoyment.
d) The improvement in myself.
e) Membership of a group.
f) Good trainer.
g) Fear of becoming unfit again.
h) Upward spiral of well-being.
i) Group session and the pub.
j) Husband/wife.
k) Friendships.
l) Not to let group down.
m) Conviction that I could improve further.
n) Enthusiasm.
o) Knowing it was good for me.
p) £100.

Those of the anaerobic group were rather similar:
a) Commitment.
b) Hope to get fitter.

c) Feeling better.
d) Determination.
e) Feeling of progress.
f) Didn't want to let organisers down.
g) Enjoyment.
h) Hate to give up once started.
i) Wanted to know how body had changed after one year.
j) Desire not to fail.
k) Didn't want to let group down.
l) Because of husband/wife.
m) £100.
n) Good instructor.
o) To keep aerobic or anaerobic pair intact.
p) It was doing me good.

During the course of the project it became obvious that there were several unsatisfactory details of its organisation which might be useful information for others thinking of setting up similar studies. These aspects were the purpose of the questions listed in Table 5a. Answers to these questions are given in Table 5b.

There was frequent criticism of the training programmes. This was essentially because the improvement in performance, which occurred very quickly, far exceeded the limits of the training schedules. This was less of a problem for the runners, who were able to increase their training level simply by increasing the speed or duration of their run. The anaerobic group could only increase the repetitions and became bored with the limited number of exercises very quickly. A common suggestion was that weights should have been incorporated into the schedule about halfway through the year, as well as other more varied activities including team games etc.

Another frequent criticism of the service participants received from the GETTING IN SHAPE project was that they didn't have enough encouragement and feedback from the organisers of the scientific part of the project nor the *Sunday Times*, in terms of more articles.

The testing methods used by the West London Institute of Higher Education were judged by those who felt they were entitled to do so, to be generally unpleasant, particularly the bloodletting and the breathing apparatus. They also felt that the bicycle test put them at a disadvantage because it was so different from the training they were used to, and they felt their performance was badly underrated. This complaint was given by both training groups and is very similar to that made by many patients and other healthy subjects going through the same tests at the Brompton Hospital.

The aim of the next part of the questionnaire (Table 6a) was to discover how the project had influenced the physical aspects of participants' everyday lives. Answers are listed in Table 6b.

17% of the participants were smokers at the beginning of the study (Fig. 2 and Table 6b). Of those who responded, more than half reduced their smoking, i.e. 18% decreased the number of cigarettes they smoked in a day and 41% stopped altogether. This response was twice as marked in the anaerobes as in the aerobes. This may well account for much of the reduction in inaccessible gas volume (TLC – VA) that was seen as training progressed.

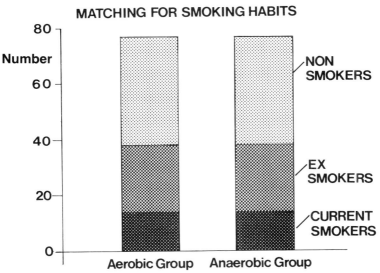

Figure 2   A histogram of smoking habits in the aerobic and anaerobic group to show the degree of matching.

39% of the respondents believed the year's training had improved the quality of their sleep. Much the same number (45.5%) believed it had changed their eating habits. The women tended to report eating less, particularly less sugar and 'stodge', and the men reported eating more (of everything). In this regard, there was no difference between the two groups. Alcohol consumption was not affected as often (19%). Most of these respondents noted a reduction but five of them recorded increases (because they could tolerate more as they became fitter).

About 40% of the respondents observed an increase in stamina. None reported a decrease. In this respect there were no differences between aerobes and anaerobes or men and women. Over half of the respondents (55%) sensed an increase in their mental alertness at work. None felt a decrease. Just under half of the respondents reported they had lost weight. Most of these were aerobes. Measurements at the time of exercise tests show weight changes were usually small (Figs. 3 and 4). Those who felt they had lost weight reported the site of loss (in order of descending frequency) as follows:

AEROBIC

a) Waist.
b) Thighs/bottom.
c) Upper part of body.
d)

ANAEROBIC

Waist.
Bottom.
Thighs.
Upper part of body.

Changes in physical appearance were mostly related to weight loss and an increase in muscle tone. The descriptions of how they felt their appearances had changed were as follows:

AEROBIC

FEMALES

a) Firmer thighs and bottom.
b) Flatter stomach.
c) Generally improved.
d) Less flabby.
e) Slimmer.
f)

MALES

General improvement.
Smaller waist.
Toned-up leg muscles.
Better posture.
Thinner.
Fatter.

ANAEROBIC

FEMALES

a) Generally better shape.
b) Firmer arms and legs.
c) Better posture.
d) Thicker waist.
e) Side of thighs thinner.
f) Less flabby.

MALES

Increased muscle.
Less beer gut.
More youthful.
More upright.
Chest bigger.
Smaller waist and bottom.

The most important aim of the questionnaire was to discover whether the year's training had altered the quality of the participants' lives and if so, how.

The questions we used to explore this aspect of the project are listed in Table 7a. People's responses are summarised in Table 7b. Four out of five of the respondents wished to continue physical training at the same or an increased level after the project had ended. This was as true of aerobes as anaerobes. Most of the anaerobes were keen to transfer to aerobic exercise, but some, particularly women, wished to do a mixture of both. A

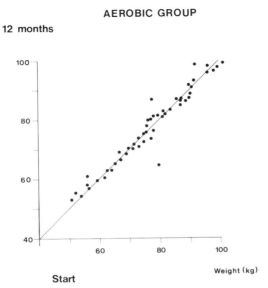

Figure 3   A plot of weight at the start and at 12 months in the aerobic group.

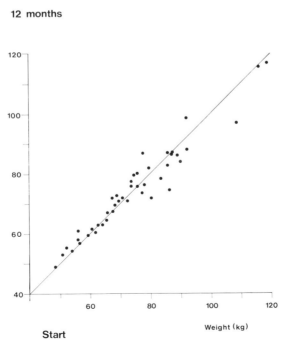

Figure 4   A plot of weight at the start and at 12 months in the anaerobic group.

small number of aerobes (7%) wished to transfer in the opposite direction. Most respondents (74%), wanted to continue with group training and also felt happy to participate in a similar study again (83%).

Most respondents attached more importance to health and physical *stamina* than strength or appearance (Table 7b). They found that the year's training had improved their stamina (sometimes dramatically), and secondly their health, then their body shape, physical strength and lastly facial appearance. Nine out of ten (92%) felt the project had been worth their investment of £100.

Asked to identify whether, and if so how, the project had done them any good, the free-style response indicates that all but one aerobe and six anaerobes felt it had. These replies and those to the subsequent (and last) two demands of the questionnaire are the crux of the study, in that they show that most people benefited to an extent that exceeded expectations and could not be divined from the exercise tests or lung-function studies. Because they are so important, we have listed these replies more or less verbatim, in Appendix 2. If any reader doubts 'the case for exercise' they should look at that list, which gives compelling evidence of the way it changed the quality of these people's lives.

DISCUSSION

In essence, this study provides data that may help to answer several questions. It also poses a fresh one. The questions it may help to answer are these:

Are present standards for normal lung-function tests appropriate to the local population at this time? The standards we and many other centres use are based on populations from elsewhere at other times. These population characteristics show geographical variations that also change with time. On the other hand, the population selected by the advertisement for this study is not typical of the people of London as a whole, in that the present group is taller, heavier, more affluent, and probably less fit but more health conscious than the population at large. Nevertheless, they are the only recent, appropriately-aged reference population we have, and they suggest we need to modify some standards slightly but significantly. They also answer an unfulfilled need for a standard of accessible lung volume (VA). The shortfall of VA on total lung capacity forms the inaccessible gas volume or volume of lung which is 'out of service'. This appears to be some 13% of the whole.

Are present standards for normal responses to progressive exercise tests appropriate to the local population at this time? Yes, it seems so, in the sense that we deliberately recruited a group of unfit people who began slightly below par, and finished with a group of untypically active people who were, on average, slightly above par.

Did the change in physical status of the subjects with training modify their lung-function characteristics at all? Yes, but only slightly, and according to need, in that the biggest changes are seen in those beginning with the lowest values, i.e. the response is roughly proportionate to need, but the changes are slight. The inaccessible gas volume (TLC − VA) appears to be distinctly sensitive to physical training.

Did the training schedules used here have any effect on people's aerobic capacity? Yes, the anaerobes improved by an average of 7% and the aerobes by an average of 14%.

Did the training schedules used here have any effect on people's 'well-being'? Yes, considerable subjective benefits of the programme were felt by almost all the participants and, to the extent that the improvements can be equated, seemed to be out of all proportion to the modest increases in aerobic capacity and lung function.

Is it possible to identify who will benefit from training, and who will not? That depends on the definition of benefit. Certainly, the improvements in aerobic capacity were roughly proportional to the initial shortfall in capacity relative to predicted values. People below predicted levels improved their capacity. Those above did not, even élite athletes.

Is it possible to rank the two methods of training? Yes, but with caution. It is foolish to improve at tennis by practising the piano. Similarly with physical training. If its purpose is to improve aerobic capacity then, not surprisingly, aerobic training is more effective than anaerobic training. It is also less boring.

The fresh question posed by the study is this: **Does aerobic capacity reflect physical fitness?** The answer to this is by no means sure. Aerobic capacity is a physical characteristic that is quite reproducible ($\pm 7.5\%$) in healthy individuals. It is also, very certainly, greatly reduced in disease (Fig. 5). However, the normal range of values in a group of people of the same age, sex and body size is $\pm 40\%$, which leaves a very wide interval (from 140% down to 60%) through which an individual's aerobic capacity could slide before being found abnormal on first inspection. Serial testing would, of course, reveal this trend, but at

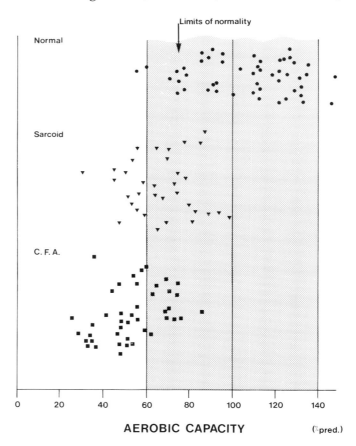

Figure 5   Observations on the symptom-limited maximum oxygen consumption of three groups of people: a) 34 healthy subjects, b) 39 patients with proven pulmonary sarcoidosis, and c) 41 patients with proven cryptogenic fibrosing alveolitis. Note how many of the patients have undoubtedly reduced aerobic capacities but are still within the normal range.

increased cost in time and money to subject and laboratory. More importantly, physical fitness is not measurable until defined. Defined as aerobic capacity it can be measured. Defined as physical well-being it cannot, although the subjective reports recorded here indicate that the latter changes in a more marked way than does aerobic capacity. This may lie at the root of the difficulty experienced in clinical medicine, where it is sometimes, even often, difficult to relate changes in doctor's or patient's impression of clinical state to measured responses to conventional progressive exercise tests. Are we measuring the right things and if not what should we be measuring?

Clinical exercise tests are usually, but not always, demanded with a purpose: to detect depression of the S-T segment (one of several peaks in each heartbeat) of the ECG in suspected ischaemic heart disease; to reveal broncho-constriction in exercise-induced asthma; to uncover desaturation of arterial blood in damage to the pulmonary capillary bed. For these purposes the exercise tests are appropriate, although as far as the lung is concerned there is some evidence that they can be replaced by simpler procedures e.g. cold air inhalation for exercise-induced asthma, or measurements of TLCO at rest for restrictive lung disease. They are also apposite, as shown here, for identifying those people likely to benefit from physical training, for motivating them and for providing some evidence of their progress. They seem poor reflectors, however, of the quality of people's daily lives. The element they seem to ignore is that of stamina. Perhaps this is the element that participants and patients sense and measurers miss. What we need is some *brief*, *objective* test of this.

PRINCIPAL CONCLUSION

The principal conclusion of the study must be the message contained in Appendix 2, i.e. when a group of self-admittedly sedentary people take on a programme of physical training they find it transforms their lives, giving them alertness, stamina and the resource to cope with everyday life more easily than before.

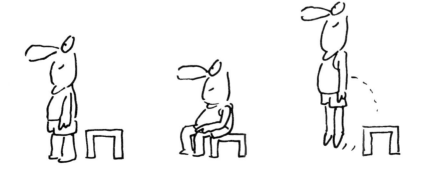

Table 1a

PRE-PROJECT CONDITION

Q.1. How did you feel, physically, before the project?

Q.2. Would you say you were: a) Very fit
                                       b) Moderately fit
                                       c) Average
                                       d) Slightly unfit
                                       e) Very unfit

Q.3. How long was it since you took any form of regular exercise of moderate intensity? e.g. twenty minutes – enough to make you out of breath – three times a week:

                                a) Less than 6 months
                                b) 6 months to 1 year
                                c) 1–2 years
                                d) 2–5 years
                                e) 5–10 years
                                f) 10–20 years

Please describe any exercise you have done since school or college:

Q.4. Did you do sports/PE at school?   Y/N

Q.5. How many of the options open to you were individual activities rather than team games?

                                a) All
                                b) Most
                                c) Half and half
                                d) Few
                                e) None

Q.6. Did you enjoy sports generally?   Y/N

Q.7. If so, which were your favourite activities?

Q.8. Did you enjoy serious competition, friendly competition, or merely playing for pleasure?

Q.9. Do you think your school PE has influenced your physical activity since then?

                                                          Yes/No/Uncertain

If Yes, has it been: a) Positive
                                        b) Negative

Table 1b

PRE-PROJECT CONDITION – RESPONSES

QUESTIONS   RESPONSES

N.B. Not all respondents answered every question.

Q.1.	(General physical condition)		See text
Q.2.	(Felt)	a) Very fit	1%
		b) Moderately fit	7%
		c) Average	25%
		d) Slightly unfit	45%
		e) Very unfit	22%
Q.3.	(Last regular exercise)		
		a) Less than 6 months	3%
		b) 6 months to 1 year	7%
		c) 1–2 years	3%
		d) 2–5 years	10%
		e) 5–10 years	24%
		f) 10–20 years	54%
		g) Never	4%
	(Description of exercise)		See text
Q.4.	(School sports)	a) Yes	96%
		b) No	4%
Q.5.	(Individual or team games)		
		a) All	4%
		b) Mostly	5%
		c) Half and half	32%
		d) Few	44%
		e) None	15%
Q.6.	(Enjoy sports)	a) Yes	73%
		b) No	26%
Q.7.	(Favourite activities)		See text
Q.8.	(Enjoy)	a) Serious competition	32%
		b) Friendly competition	34%
		c) Pleasure	22%
Q.9.	(PE influence activity)		
		a) Yes	51%
		b) No	49%
	(If yes)	a) Positive	50%
		b) Negative	50%

Table 2a

MOTIVATION

Q.1.   Before reading the advertisement did you think there was any particular interest in physical activity in:
   a) this country
   b) another country

Q.2.   If so, did it influence your decision to take any action?

Q.3.   If yes, did the influence come from this country or abroad?

Q.4.   Did any other sporting connection influence you?

Q.5.   Did you read the *Sunday Times* advertisement yourself?

   Did the advertisement bring the question of physical fitness to your attention?

Q.6.   Below are listed some possible motives for participating in the study. Please indicate below the importance of each one to you:

	VERY IMP	FAIRLY IMP	NOT IMP	DON'T KNOW
a) Reducing the risk of heart disease				
b) Improving general health				
c) Loss of weight				
d) Improving general appearance				
e) Publicity				
f) Meeting people				
g) Exercising in a group rather than by yourself				
h) Competing against your own standard				
i) Using supervised exercise programme				
j) Competing with others				

Q.7.   Before the study began, if asked the question:
   'Do you think the exercise regimes being used will improve your GENERAL fitness?' Would you have said:

   1) AEROBIC – Yes / Not Sure / No
   2) ANAEROBIC – Yes / Not Sure / No

Table 2b

MOTIVATION – RESPONSES

QUESTIONS		RESPONSES		
		BOTH	AEROBES	ANAEROBES
Q.1.	(Interest in physical activity)			
	a) This country	76%	–	–
	b) Another country	61%	–	–
Q.2.	(Influence decision)			
	a) Yes	36%	–	–
	b) No	63%	–	–
Q.3.	(Source of influence)			
	a) This country	74%	–	–
	b) Abroad	26%	–	–
Q.4.	(Other connection)			
	a) Yes	15%	–	–
	b) No	85%	–	–
Q.5.	(Read advertisement)			
	a) Yes	94%	–	–
	b) No	6%	–	–
	(Attention to physical fitness)			
	a) Yes	76%	–	–
	b) No	22%	–	–
Q.6.	(Motives)			
	a) Heart disease risk			
	a) Very important	43%	–	–
	b) Fairly important	37%	–	–
	c) Not important	20%	–	–
	b) General health			
	a) Very important	79%	–	–
	b) Fairly important	21%	–	–
	c) Not important	0%	–	–
	c) Weight loss			
	a) Very important	37%	–	–
	b) Fairly important	30%	–	–
	c) Not important	33%	–	–
	d) General appearance			
	a) Very important	29%	–	–
	b) Fairly important	45%	–	–
	c) Not important	27%	–	–
	e) Publicity			
	a) Very important	1%	–	–
	b) Fairly important	6%	–	–
	c) Not important	93%	–	–
	f) Meeting people			
	a) Very important	8%	–	–
	b) Fairly important	38%	–	–
	c) Not important	54%	–	–
	g) Group exercise			
	a) Very important	35%	–	–
	b) Fairly important	40%	–	–
	c) Not important	25%	–	–

h) Self competition				
a) Very important	17%	–	–	
b) Fairly important	54%	–	–	
c) Not important	29%	–	–	
i) Supervised exercise				
a) Very important	55%	–	–	
b) Fairly important	38%	–	–	
c) Not important	7%	–	–	
j) Competition				
a) Very important	4%	–	–	
b) Fairly important	22%	–	–	
c) Not important	75%	–	–	

Q.7.   (Regimes improve GENERAL fitness)

a) Yes	–	88%	67%
b) Not sure	–	12%	33%

Table 3a
EXPECTATIONS OF TRAINING

Q.1.   What influenced your choice between aerobic and anaerobic training?

Q.2.   Did you expect to lose weight?   Yes / No / Don't know

Q.3.   Did you think your chance of getting into the group of your choice was:

                  a) Very good
                  b) Fairly good
                  c) Even
                  d) Fairly poor
                  e) Very poor
                  f) Don't know

Q.4.   Did you expect to enjoy your chosen method of exercise:

                  a) A great deal
                  b) Fairly well
                  c) Unsure
                  d) Not a great deal
                  e) Not at all

Table 3b
EXPECTATIONS OF TRAINING – RESPONSES

QUESTIONS		RESPONSES		
		BOTH	AEROBES	ANAEROBES
Q.1.	(Influence on choice)	See text	–	–
Q.2.	(Weight loss expectation)			
	a) Yes	66%	–	–
	b) No	25%	–	–
	c) Don't know	8%	–	–

Q.3. (Chance of group of choice)

a) Very good	–	4%	9%
b) Fairly good	–	22%	20%
c) Even	–	8%	13%
d) Fairly poor	–	16%	27%
e) Very poor	–	10%	7%
f) Don't know	–	18%	25%

Q.4. (Enjoy chosen method of exercise)

a) A great deal	–	15%	23%
b) Fairly well	–	35%	44%
c) Unsure	–	19%	21%
d) Not a great deal	–	25%	9%
e) Not at all	–	6%	4%

Table 4a

IMPACT OF TRAINING

Q.1. Was the first training session:
- a) Very easy
- b) Easy
- c) Between b) & e)
- d) Hard
- e) Very hard

Q.2. Was the first training session:
- a) Very enjoyable
- b) Enjoyable
- c) Indifferent
- d) Not enjoyable
- e) Unpleasant

Q.3. During the rest of the week did you usually exercise:
- a) On your own
- b) With a friend/relative – not participating
- c) With another participant

How many workout sessions did you complete on average a week?

If sessions were missed was it mostly due to:
- a) Lack of time
- b) Lack of motivation
- c) Others

Q.4. Was the training during the week:
- a) Easier
- b) Same
- c) Harder

to complete than the group sessions?

Q.5. Did you prefer to exercise in the morning or evening?

Q.6. (WOMEN AEROBICS)
Did you ever run alone in the dark?   Y/N

Q.7. Did you feel safe running on your own in the dark?   Y/N
Did you feel safe running on your own in the daylight?   Y/N

Q.8. Did you at any time seriously consider withdrawing from the project?   Y/N

Q.9.   Was there a competitive spirit in your group? Yes / No / Don't know

Q.10. For you personally, was this: a) Good
                                       b) Indifferent
                                       c) Bad

Q.11. Did your family/friends show any reaction to your involvement in
       the project?   Y/N

Q.12. If yes, was it: a) Positive   b) Neutral   c) Negative

Q.13. Did you usually stay for a drink with the group afterwards?
                           a) Always   b) Most of the time
                           c) Sometimes   d) Never

Q.14. Did you enjoy the social aspects of the project? Yes / No / Uncertain

Q.15. What was the main thing that kept you going until the end of the
       year?

Table 4b

IMPACT OF TRAINING – RESPONSES

QUESTIONS		RESPONSES	
	BOTH	AEROBES	ANAEROBES
Q.1. (First session)			
a) Very easy	–	19%	49%
b) Easy	–	23%	19%
c) Between b) & e)	–	21%	14%
d) Hard	–	13%	9%
e) Very hard	–	25%	9%
Q.2. (First session)			
a) Very enjoyable	–	14%	13%
b) Enjoyable	–	55%	57%
c) Indifferent	–	18%	16%
d) Not enjoyable	–	10%	11%
e) Unpleasant	–	2%	4%
Q.3. (Usually exercise)			
a) On your own	–	76%	88%
b) With a friend/relative	–	10%	5%
c) With another participant		14%	7%
(No. of sessions per week)			
a) 1	–	4%	0%
b) 2	–	6%	16%
c) 2–3	–	4%	8%
d) 3	–	44%	40%
e) 3–4	–	25%	14%
f) 4	–	15%	22%
g) 5	–	2%	0%
(Missed sessions)			
a) Lack of time	–	53%	47%
b) Lack of motivation	–	14%	14%
c) Others	–	33%	39%

Q.4.	(Training during week)					
	a) Easier (than in group)	–	10%		25%	
	b) Same	–	29%		15%	
	c) Harder	–	61%		60%	
Q.5.	(Prefer to exercise)					
	a) Morning	–	33%		47%	
	b) Evening	–	57%		51%	
	c) Both	–	10%		2%	
Q.6.	(WOMEN AEROBICS) (Run alone in dark)					
	a) Yes	–	74%		–	
	b) No	–	26%		–	
Q.7.	(Safe in dark)					
	a) Yes	–	38%		–	
	b) No	–	57%		–	
	c) No reply	–	5%		–	
	(Safe in daylight)					
	a) Yes	–	96%		–	
	b) No	–	4%		–	
Q.8.	(Consider withdrawing)					
	a) Yes	–	16%		15%	
	b) No	–	84%		85%	
Q.9.	(Competitive spirit in group)					
	a) Yes	–	63%		44%	
	b) No	–	29%		36%	
	c) Don't know	–	8%		20%	
Q.10.	(Was this, personally)		M	F	M	F
	a) Good	–	45%	43%	67%	68%
	b) Indifferent	–	38%	7%	4%	11%
	c) Bad	–	17%	50%	29%	21%
Q.11.	(Family reaction)					
	a) Yes	–	96%		82%	
	b) No	–	4%		18%	
Q.12.	(If yes, was it)					
	a) Positive	–	81%		76%	
	b) Neutral	–	7%		9%	
	c) Negative	–	5%		7%	
Q.13.	(Drink with group)					
	a) Always	–	30%		21%	
	b) Most of the time	–	38%		33%	
	c) Sometimes	–	24%		32%	
	d) Never	–	8%		15%	
Q.14.	(Enjoy social aspects)					
	a) Yes	–	82%		66%	
	b) No	–	9%		5%	
	c) Uncertain	–	9%		29%	
Q.15.	(Main thing to keep going)				See text	

Table 5a

QUALITY OF GETTING IN SHAPE SERVICE

Q.1. Do you think that the training schedule laid out in the manuals gave you a constant increase in work load? Yes / No / Unsure

Q.2. If YES, did this keep pace with your progress?
If NO, at what stage in the programme do you think it could be changed, and how?

Q.3a. Did you think the trainers had sufficient medical 'know how' for the task they were required to undertake? Yes / No / Unsure

Q.3b. Do you think they were given adequate instruction to enable them to run the training programmes well? Yes / No / Unsure

Q.4. Did you feel that you received sufficient attention from:
1) The Brompton Yes / No / Don't know
2) The West London Institute of Higher Education Yes / No / Don't know

Q.5. Did you get any feedback concerning your progress from either of the above institutions?
1) The Brompton Yes / No / Don't know
2) The West London Institute of Higher Education
Yes / No / Don't know

Q.6. Do you think you should have got: a) Less ⎫
b) Same ⎬ feedback
c) More ⎭

Q.7. Why?

Q.8a. Were you aware of any features in the *Sunday Times* on the project throughout the year? Yes / No / Don't know

Q.8b. Do you think the coverage of the project should have been:
a) Less
b) Same
c) More

Q.9. What did you think of the methods used to measure your physical fitness at the West London?

Did you think they were:
a) Too simple
b) Just right
c) Too complex

Table 5b

QUALITY OF GETTING IN SHAPE
SERVICE – RESPONSES

QUESTIONS		RESPONSES	
	BOTH	AEROBES	ANAEROBES
Q.1. (Increased workload in schedule) a) Yes	–	82%	70%

	b) No	–	12%	30%
	c) Unsure	–	6%	0%
Q.2.	(Keep pace with progress)			
	a) Yes	–	71%	43%
	b) No	–	27%	40%
	c) Unsure	–	2%	17%
	(What stage could programme be changed)			See text
Q.3a.	(Trainers' medical 'know how')			
	a) Yes	–	55%	43%
	b) No	–	18%	25%
	c) Unsure	–	27%	32%
Q.3b.	(Trainers given enough instruction)			
	a) Yes	–	51%	39%
	b) No	–	16%	29%
	c) Unsure	–	33%	32%
Q.4.	(Enough attention from Brompton)			
	a) Yes	–	68%	86%
	b) No	–	24%	7%
	c) Don't know	–	8%	7%
	(Enough attention from WLIHE)			
	a) Yes	–	76%	89%
	b) No	–	16%	4%
	c) Don't know	–	8%	7%
Q.5.	(Feedback from Brompton)			
	a) Yes	–	57%	54%
	b) No	–	37%	41%
	c) Don't know	–	6%	5%
	(Feedback from WLIHE)			
	a) Yes	–	71%	61%
	b) No	–	27%	32%
	c) Don't know	–	2%	7%
Q.6.	(Received feedback)			
	a) Less	–	0%	0%
	b) Same	–	27%	17%
	c) More	–	73%	83%
Q.7.	(Why?)			See text
Q.8a.	(Awareness of *Sunday Times* features)			
	a) Yes	–	92%	93%
	b) No	–	8%	7%
	c) Don't know	–	0%	0%
Q.8b.	(Project coverage)			
	a) Less	–	0%	2%
	b) Same	–	16%	22%
	c) More	–	84%	76%
Q.9.	(WLIHE methods)			
	a) Too simple	–	19%	14%
	b) Just right	–	81%	67%
	c) Too complex	–	0%	19%

Table 6a

PHYSICAL CHANGES

Q.1.   Did you smoke at the beginning of the project?
Yes / No / Ex-smoker

Q.2.   Has your smoking: a) Increased
          b) Stayed the same
          c) Decreased
          d) Stopped

Q.3a. Has the training affected the quality of your sleep?

Q.3b. If YES, how?

Q.4a. Has the training altered your eating habits?
Yes / No / Don't know

Q.4b. If YES, how?

Q.5a. Has the training altered your alcohol consumption?
Yes / No / Don't know

Q.5b. If YES, how?

Q.6.   Has your daily physical stamina: a) Stayed the same
               b) Decreased
               c) Increased
               d) Don't know

Q.7.   Has your mental alertness at work: a) Stayed the same
               b) Decreased
               c) Increased

Q.8a. Have you lost weight over the year?

Q.8b. Was it: a) Less than 5 lb
      b) 5–7 lb
      c) 7–10 lb
      d) 10–14 lb
      e) 1–2 stone
      f) More

Q.8c. Where do you feel most of the weight has gone from:
            a) Upper part of your body
            b) Waist
            c) Legs and thighs
            d) Bottom
            e) N/A

Q.9a. Have you noticed any change in your physical appearance over the year? Yes / No

Q.9b. If YES, please describe:

Table 6b

PHYSICAL CHANGES – RESPONSES

QUESTIONS		BOTH	AEROBES	ANAEROBES
RESPONSES				
Q.1.	(Smoke at start)			
	a) Yes	–	15%	18%
	b) No	–	68%	52%
	c) Ex-smoker	–	17%	30%
Q.2.	(Has smoking)			
	a) Increased	–	0%	0%
	b) Stayed the same	–	57%	30%
	c) Decreased	–	14%	20%
	d) Stopped	–	29%	50%
Q.3a.	(Sleep affected)			
	a) Yes	–	49%	31%
	b) No	–	13%	3%
	c) Don't know	–	38%	66%
Q.3b.	(If YES, how)			See text
Q.4a.	(Changed eating habits)			
	a) Yes	–	50%	41%
	b) No	–	42%	54%
	c) Don't know	–	8%	5%
Q.4b.	(If YES, how)			See text
Q.5a.	(Changed alcohol consumption)			
	a) Yes	–	26%	12%
	b) No	–	70%	86%
	c) Don't know	–	4%	2%
Q.5b.	(If YES, how)			See text
Q.6.	(Daily physical stamina)			
	a) Stayed the same	–	21%	24%
	b) Decreased	–	0%	0%
	c) Increased	–	34%	41%
	d) Don't know	–	4%	2%
Q.7.	(Mental alertness at work)			
	a) Stayed the same	–	47%	43%
	b) Decreased	–	0%	0%
	c) Increased	–	53%	57%
Q.8a.	(Weight loss)			
	a) Yes	–	65%	26%
	b) No	–	35%	74%
Q.8b.	(Was it . . .)			
	a) Less than 5 lb	–	26%	12%
	b) 5–7 lb	–	27%	44%
	c) 7–10 lb	–	22%	13%
	d) 10–14 lb	–	15%	19%

e) 1–2 stone	–	11%	6%
f) More	–	0%	6%

Q.8c. (Most weight gone from . . .)

a) Upper part of body	–	9%	9%
b) Waist	–	36%	31%
c) Legs and thighs	–	19%	10%
d) Bottom	–	19%	17%
e) N/A	–	11%	17%

Q.9a. (Change in physical appearance over year)   See text

Q.9b. (If YES, describe)   See text

Table 7a

OVERALL REACTION

Q.1. Would you like to continue exercising: a) Less often
b) Same amount
c) More often
d) Not at all
e) Don't know

Q.2. Would you continue with the same type of exercise as you have been:
a) Yes
b) Don't know
c) No

Q.3. If NO, please specify the alternative you would prefer.
AEROBICS – Would you like to try doing the anaerobic exercises?

Q.4. Would you prefer to exercise: a) In a group
b) Alone
c) With one or two people

Q.5. Would you participate in a study of this kind again?
Yes / No / Unsure

Q.6. Please indicate the extent to which each of the following concern you:

	NOT IMPORTANT	FAIRLY IMPORTANT	VERY IMPORTANT
a) Health			
b) Facial appearance			
c) Body shape			
d) Physical stamina			
e) Physical strength			

Q.7. Which of the following has improved over the year:
a) Health
b) Facial appearance
c) Body shape
d) Physical stamina
e) Physical strength
f) None have
g) Other
(Please indicate on the scale above the size of the improvement)
Rating 1–6: 1 = low.

Q.8. Do you think your participation in the project was worth £100 to you?   Yes / No / Uncertain

Q.9. Do you think it has done you any good? Please explain.

Q.10. Has your awareness of how your body looks altered at all?
        If YES, is your awareness: a) Less   b) Same   c) More

Q.11. Do you feel any different now compared with the start of the project?   Yes / No
        Please would you describe this feeling.

Q.12. Do you notice any difference in your ability to cope with the usual physical demands of your daily life?

Table 7b

OVERALL REACTION – RESPONSES

QUESTIONS		BOTH	RESPONSES AEROBES	ANAEROBES
Q.1.	(Continue exercise)			
	a) Less often	–	18%	10%
	b) Same amount	–	49%	57%
	c) More often	–	31%	31%
	d) Not at all	–	2%	2%
	e) Don't know	–	0%	0%
Q.2.	(Same exercise)			
	a) Yes	–	81%	43%
	b) Don't know	–	15%	52%
	c) No	–	4%	5%
Q.3.	(If no, preferences)			See text
Q.4.	(Prefer to exercise)			
	a) In a group	–	65%	82%
	b) Alone	–	9%	8%
	c) With one or two people	–	26%	10%
Q.5.	(Take part again)			
	a) Yes	–	88%	77%
	b) No	–	0%	7%
	c) Unsure	–	12%	16%
Q.6.	(Importance of:)			
	a) Health			
	a) Not important	0%	–	–
	b) Fairly important	11%	–	–
	c) Very important	89%	–	–
	b) Facial appearance			
	a) Not important	16%	–	–
	b) Fairly important	59%	–	–
	c) Very important	25%	–	–
	c) Body shape			
	a) Not important	4%	–	–
	b) Fairly important	54%	–	–
	c) Very important	42%	–	–

d)	Physical stamina			
	a) Not important	0%	–	–
	b) Fairly important	33%	–	–
	c) Very important	67%	–	–
e)	Physical strength			
	a) Not important	15%	–	–
	b) Fairly important	56%	–	–
	c) Very important	29%	–	–
Q.7.	(Improved over the year)			
	a) Health	–	30%	43%
	b) Facial appearance	–	17%	24%
	c) Body shape	–	33%	39%
	d) Physical stamina	–	41%	51%
	e) Physical strength	–	22%	40%
	f) None have	–	3%	8%
	g) Other	–	1%	1%
Q.8.	(Worth £100)			
	a) Yes	–	88%	96%
	b) No	–	4%	2%
	c) Uncertain	–	8%	2%
Q.9.	(Explain any good of project)			See text
Q.10.	(Altered awareness of body)			
	a) Less	–	5%	0%
	b) Same	–	48%	53%
	c) More	–	48%	47%
Q.11.	(Feel different)			
	a) Yes	–	89%	79%
	b) No	–	11%	21%
Q.12.	(Notice change in ability to cope with demands)			See text

APPENDIX 2

We have included everybody's comments more or less verbatim, only excluding those remarks that might identify people easily to each other. None of the excluded comments alter the balance of the message given here.

AEROBES

'In the summer – which was halfway into the programme – I felt much fitter. However, I find, being asthmatic, the cold affects my breathing badly.'

'I feel so much younger and logical and self-confident, fitter and healthier.'

'Much happier with my shape, healthier and more alert.'

'My physical, mental and emotional health have all improved uniformly. I have a greater knowledge of my own ability and am more prepared to take risks and keep going when it gets difficult in all three fields.'

'My body now feels more part of me – more alive – more friend than enemy. If I can learn to run a marathon at forty-four, then I can have a go at most things. I feel as if the ageing process has been reversed.'

'Apart from the days I have been running long distances, I do not seem to tire physically any more. My menstrual cycle is less obstructive to life, being of short duration and light. This I put down to tighter, fitter muscles. Having children has damaged many muscles, but this weakness is much less apparent.'

'I have learnt a lot about myself, some good, some bad. I have never been neurotic, but I now no longer seem to worry about anything (not always a good thing, I'm sure).'

'I no longer feel like a fat slob (whether I should is another matter) even though my weight is unchanged. I still want to lose weight – to make the running easier, though, rather than to improve my appearance.'

'Much more alive most of the time.'

'I now feel very fit.'

'I now try to persuade others to take up exercise.'

'I now seem to be able to deal with daily problems easier and I similarly hope I will be able to complete the London Marathon on 13th May. Twelve months ago according to my diary, I was pleased to stop after seven minutes.'

'I am able to cope with stress much better. Lost a stone in weight, 1" off my waist and clothes that fitted me ten years ago (i.e. same size) still fit.

'Problems do not appear as difficult. Able to sustain rigorous exercise for much longer periods and not get so tired either.'

'Definitely, life's challenge is enjoyed.'

'All round improvements.'

'Made me much more conscious of how to exercise sensibly.'

'Great confidence booster (knowing improvement made).'

'Willing to tackle almost anything – except to climb Nelson's column.'

'It has given me enthusiasm to take up other physical activities and in general lead a more active life.'

'More balanced lifestyle. Less aggressive, calmer. Turning to sports or physical activities when under pressure rather than food or drink.'

'I tire less easily and walk or run to venues rather than drive from door to door.'

'I am more motivated towards taking regular exercise, which I feel has benefited me as a discipline. The project helped me through what were probably the most difficult years of my life to date, both emotionally and physically.'

'I am aware that I have more stamina, am more alert, and have more of a sense of well-being generally. I just wish that the weight would come off and that I could sleep better!'

'Coping better than before with less effort.'

'I feel much healthier and fitter.'

'I feel more confident and have a feeling of well-being.'

'Much less stressful.'

'Apart from previously mentioned benefits, I think better, relate better, and make and stick to decisions better.'

'More positive.'

'Daily life is more easy.'

'General improved feeling of physical confidence and mental confidence to a degree.'

'More stamina.'

'I'm able to run quite long distances and have an urge to do a marathon, but for the time being I've stopped running.'

'More inclined to exercise, more vigorous (especially in the mornings). Greater stamina.'

'I can now do things I couldn't do a year ago.'

'I feel fitter and able to do physical exercises etc. that I couldn't do a year ago and no longer feel afraid of exercising.'

'Had to give up just at end of year because of recurring medical problems with knees. This, plus bout of anaemia and bout of bronchitis (both first time) meant that I started three times! So never really climbed more than first hill!'

'I felt more lively and had lost weight, but having had to stop jogging on GP's advice felt very disappointed and, I think, disillusioned. Have done nothing for two months now, knees and hip joints now pain-free; I've stiffened up again and am on the point of starting the anaerobic programme.'

'Although I stuck it for the year and didn't get very far, I certainly had more ''puff'' around the home etc.'

'Doing the exercise correlated with the belief that it was a good idea.'

'Much fitter, with a sense of achievement.'

'Improved.'

'I now exercise regularly, and current thinking seems to be that this is a good thing.'

'More aware of body generally, and what one does with it, and what one puts into it!'

'It has made me more aware that exercise is good and necessary.'

'Happier with myself.'

'Made new friends, boosted my self-esteem, enjoy going to and competing in races with my husband. Impressed my children.'

'Feel younger, more energetic and supple.'

'Feel much stronger, with more stamina.'

'I know I can finish a course.'

'More determined, more confident in my own ability to cope. Less willing to rely on other people or take the easy way out.'

'Yes.'

'I don't feel stagnant.'

'Increased confidence in my shape. Less concerned about always wearing make-up and hair being tidy (maybe it has made me more relaxed about my general appearance, or perhaps, scruffy!).'

'More confident and not too concerned about being in my fifties.'

'It has provided a hobby, something to take my mind off work which is very important to me and sometimes looms too large in my life. I'm devoting time to myself for a change.'

'More confident.'

'I still react in the same way, waking early and worrying. I had hoped that the project would help me overcome this – it hasn't.'

'On a positive note, my energy level is higher.'

'I learnt to compete at something sporting. I learnt to pace myself, to know even when I felt ghastly, if I kept going I'd eventually die or feel much better.'

'Stronger physically and mentally and physically braver.'

'I think a twelve-month period of commitment to regular exercise is long enough both to convince one it is worthwhile and to learn the habit of actually getting out and doing it.'

'I feel younger and I have no doubt that my transition into middle-age will be much easier and I will stay fit and healthy (bombs and AIDS permitting) into my sixties with the help of regular exercise, which I am sure I will now keep up.'

'Obviously, it is good to have strengthened heart and lungs. General sense of well-being and increased self-confidence, most of all my outlook on life has changed, I feel twenty years younger.'

'Younger outlook, I enjoy physical exertion whereas before I kept it to the minimum.'

'It has made me aware of the need for constant exercise to assist my health and appearance.'

'A general feeling of better appearance (I hope it shows) and a happier manner (i.e. I don't go around snapping people's heads off).'

'I definitely feel I have a greater ability to cope, but whether this lasts remains to be seen! Obviously, I must keep up the exercise to avoid slipping back. I certainly intend to do so but time will tell, for without group spirit it is very hard.'

'It got me off my bum. I feel better. Will continue with some of my group, still keen.'

'Daily life is easier.'

'Given me an outlet from stress of work other than alcohol.'

'More willing to undertake physical tasks.'

'Everything from readiness to climb stairs to willingness to bend down and unbolt a door.'

'Am determined to carry on some form of regular exercise. Understand, I think, my body a little better.'

'I think my lung function has improved. Disappointed that through injury at end of training (last six weeks) end tests showed no improvement over middle tests.'

'I have been more positive in making decisions (perhaps aggressive). My life style has improved because I pay more attention to what is going on around me, and my eating habits are more extensive.'

'I feel fitter and more alive.'

'Yes, I can cope a lot better.'

'Don't seem to get migraine (stress) headaches as used to; and resting pulse gone from 88 to less than 60.'

'Knew I was fat before!'

'Given me confidence that improvements can be achieved.'

'A sense of confidence and well-being (not necessarily in-fluenced by GIS. I was undertaking a fairly rigorous appraisal of my attitudes to life prior (to the project). I am not sure how much GIS helped).'

ANAEROBES

'It has done considerable damage.'

'Yes, though my participation tailed off because of travelling and becoming rather bored, anything that gets the machine working feels good. Attempting the anaerobic was interesting.'

'Somewhat less fatigue; would have been more improvement if I hadn't tailed off.'

'Yes, increased fitness must do some good. I feel much better than I did when I started.'

'More positive, more energetic, more healthy, fewer colds, better able to handle stress.'

'Yes, I find it easier. When one's physical health improves, one's mental and emotional health must also improve. The three are too closely related not to affect each other.'

'Feeling more confident and competent in my body. "Standing my ground." Occasionally after exercise a feeling of euphoria. Two examples: I used to be nervous of becoming breathless because I didn't know what the consequences would be. I'd avoid running for buses – fear I couldn't catch my breath again. Now I know I can recover quickly; and I've always enjoyed swimming but never tried more than a few lengths at a time. Now I can swim thirty plus (though I don't often have time) without much strain.'

'Has launched me on a long-term programme of exercise. Had tried for years to take this up but nothing else had succeeded in maintaining commitment.'

'After taking up weight training, I began to feel fitter, less tired, and had a slightly heightened sense of well-being.'

'It has done me good. I am less of a hypochondriac and the little aches and pains have disappeared – were they ever there?'

'I am more aware of my body and realise that its well-being depends on me. I shall now follow the "prevention is better than cure" philosophy.'

'I stuck to the programme for six months and found an optimum level of fitness. I enjoy being fit.'

'I am happier with the way I am.'

'I am confirmed in my knowledge that I enjoy exercise in any form.'

'I know I cope best when I'm physically fit, but I find it difficult to find the time to do the exercise. A particular commitment is very useful.'

'I have enjoyed the social aspects of the group involvement and I have found it beneficial to be able to mix with people of many different types and ages. I have become aware that goals are very important to me.'

'It made me think of health and fitness; eliminated my back and neck aches which were of very long standing; discovered I was fitter than I thought.'

'I have enjoyed the year and the company of the eight to ten die-hards who met regularly right till the end.'

'I feel fitter, particularly circulation. I feel the cold less and my ankles don't swell any more.'

'Fitter and sense of achievement having started the course.'

'It has given me the discipline to stick at exercising, something I never had before.'

'A little more relaxed, a little more energy.'

'Want to continue to exercise and expand sporting interests.'

'Can definitely walk briskly for longer and get less tired. Recovery from exercise or physical activity is quicker.'

'Has improved own self-image. Helped me at a crucial point in life to recapture feeling of physical health that was attained in sporting days.'

'An inward feeling of being good.'

'Not much! Certainly I don't notice it subjectively.'

'I still get utterly exhausted doing housework or climbing stairs and step ladders all day long. Training does not seem to be any use except for what you are trained to do! But perhaps I should now have been in poor health if I hadn't exercised. I fear my answers seem rather negative. I am very disappointed not to feel lighter of step, and indeed, lighter in weight. Yet I now have rock-solid thighs and rock-solid trunk (so much so that my already large waist measurement has disastrously increased). I think I now "flop" more completely when relaxing, i.e. I'm less tense. But I don't sleep better, my digestive system is much the same and there isn't any other particular improvement.'

'Much better, normally would be uptight but not now.'

'I am certainly fitter and a little less of a slob!'

'More spruced up physically.'

'I have more overall stamina.'

'If nothing, it has made me realise what a long-term effort keeping healthy is. You can't get fit in a month; on the other hand, if you're fairly consistent, you can have some weeks off.'

'I feel more in charge of my body.'

'I have more stamina. If I do get tired, I can rest, or have a nap and feel ready to continue. Even doing anaerobics, I can run for the bus and recover more quickly. I get restless now if I've got nothing to do.'

'Helped me understand fitness and exercise in a more subjective way (as a student including exercise physiology in my finals!).'

'Stronger and less likely to get out of breath running up four flights of stairs at college.'

'Suffer from bad back, wrists, neck, knees. Don't know if they have been aggravated by exercise, or whether they would have deteriorated anyway.'

'It has made me more aware of how unfit I was and how fit I could be.'

'I have almost become hooked on the idea that physical fitness alters your attitudes to almost everything – food, play, work, sex, tolerance of others – all to the benefit of oneself and friends.'

'I am less bad-tempered and tired and more tolerant, but I am also more selfish. I must have time to do the things I want to do and I have more energy and fun doing them, so God help anyone who gets in my way!!!'

'It has made me more aware of keeping fit than I was. I now anticipate exercising indefinitely, which I shouldn't have considered before.'

'I believe stamina has improved.'

'Has convinced me of need to stay fit, I feel better for it. Previously unconvinced of personal benefits.'

'Get less tired.'

'It has made me more aware of exercise generally and its benefits if done on a consistent basis.'

'I am more aware of my general health through visits to Brompton Hospital.'

'Made me more aware of the importance of exercise, not just as a means of prolonging life, but as a means of improving current quality of life.'

'More physically confident.'

'I recover from tiredness more quickly.'

'It has changed my life completely.'

'I feel fit, energetic, mentally alert, more assertive, self-confident. Tremendous stamina, I've become much more selfish for myself (caring of myself).'

'I can, having decided to do something, do it so much more effortlessly. Molehills are no longer mountains. Life has perspective again.'

'Apart from physical fitness, my mental outlook is more cheerful and optimistic.'

'I feel great.'

'Life isn't half so tiring as it used to be.'

'Much more able to cope with stress. Recovery from tiredness more rapid. Less headaches, blood pressure down.'

'Much more alive and positive about life.'

'I can cope with far more.'

'At the time, it made me feel more energetic and physically confident.'

'I do feel fitter and healthier, though I've had just as many colds. After exercise I feel able to relax more completely – less tension.'

'I feel more confident about my health – I know I'm pretty fit compared to most people my age and find that satisfying. I'm pleased to see what I can do.'

'Motivated me to an extent that I find exercise enjoyable, particularly group exercise.'

'I tire less easily.'

'I have more energy but I find I cannot sit for long and watch TV like I used to as I get too restless and have to walk around or go for a walk.'

'Better all round.'

'I can cope with stress better.'

'Physically and mentally I feel better after doing exercises.'

'I feel healthier and fitter now than I did before doing exercises.'

'I find it easier and less strenuous.'

'Though I could not go to the classes regularly, I have been doing anaerobic exercises at home mostly, not regularly. I was quite regular till December 1984, Level 24.'

'I'd just returned from a couple of weeks skiing at the start of the project and I'm certainly less fit now than then.'

'Not as beneficial as I had hoped – but that has to be because I missed quite a lot.'

'Made aware of physical limitations. Highlighted chest function.'

'Body feels more balanced. Seem able to perform physical tasks more easily. Libido improved?'

'Feel generally better and convinced as to value of regular exercise which I am determined to continue.'

'More enthusiastic re: life in general.'

'More relaxed, strength/stamina improved.'

'Younger and more able.'

'Insomuch as it has made me aware that physical activity is essential at my age (forty-four) and it has given me the incentive to carry on exercising.'

'For twenty years I have been involved in using most of my energy for my business and I now feel that I can get more enjoyment out of exercising which has "slowed me down".'

'Yes.'

'More awareness of how my body is feeling.'

'I have now adopted a regular exercise routine and above all else the project has succeeded in this.'

'It has confirmed the vague suspicion I had that I am incredibly lazy to be a fact.'

'I know I need exercise plus diet if I am going to improve – however, first I need to see a shrink to see why I have absolutely no self-discipline.'

'I am more likely to continue training with a motivation to move into jogging.'

'Much more relaxed, I think. Difficult to quantify as I find it hard to remember much of last month, let alone last year. The family tell me I am much less.'

'All in all it has been a happy and rewarding experience which I hope will continue in years to come.'

'In terms of stamina, strength and starting me on a programme of what I hope will be regular exercise.'

'Fitter and stronger.'

'I feel almost as fit as when I came out of the army in 1962.'

'I can cope with running my company which is expanding and still feel I have plenty of energy to take part in family life and sport.'

'Being fitter has helped me to work longer days without getting headaches that I suffered before the course. In fact, in the whole year I have probably only had about four headaches. If I ever sell my company I would like to be involved with sport for a living.'

'Greater stamina and some increase in muscle strength.'

'But I don't remember how I felt at the start!'

'I feel much fitter and I can now run (well, jog!)'

'It has also provided the discipline of a commitment – a good thing when one is pursuing a demanding professional life.'

'Fitter and a feeling of achievement having stuck with the course and by and large, coped with the exercise regime.'

'I got into the pain area but stuck it out. Helped mental alertness and discipline but also caused some over-positiveness (aggression?)'

'Has made exercise a lifelong commitment and way of life. Sparked interest and gave contact with others of similar inclination.'

'More physical confidence and sense of well-being. More self respect.'

'No.'

'Yes, fitness has improved self-image and better feeling, physically and mentally motivated to keep up some programme of exercise.'

'Any physical activity, even going upstairs is not such a strain, it can almost be pleasurable, the awareness that one's muscles are tackling the job with ease. Much better in all situations!'

'I felt marginally better during course and it has also shown me the level of fitness I am happy with, i.e. that I do not wish to go on to bigger and better things.'

'Less concerned about ill health in the future.'

'I still wake up tired after a night's sleep and have difficulty in keeping awake driving to work. The physical demands of my daily life are negligible without the GIS exercises.'

'It has changed my attitude: exercising used to be such an effort. Now I miss it if I don't have it.'

'My stamina has increased and I have fewer "stifled", tense feelings at work. I feel more at home in my body and get the impression my physical strength has also increased.'